HEALTH AND HUMAN DEVELOPMENT

MENTAL AND HOLISTIC HEALTH

SOME INTERNATIONAL PERSPECTIVES

HEALTH AND HUMAN DEVELOPMENT
JOAV MERRICK - SERIES EDITOR –
MEDICAL DIRECTOR, MINISTRY OF SOCIAL AFFAIRS, JERUSALEM, ISRAEL

Adolescent Behavior Research: International Perspectives
Joav Merrick and Hatim A Omar (Editors)
2007. ISBN: 1-60021-649-8

Complementary Medicine Systems: Comparison and Integration
Karl W Kratky
2008. ISBN: 978-1-60456-475-4

Pain in Children and Youth
P Schofield and J Merrick (Editors)
2008. ISBN: 978-1-60456-951-3

Obesity and Adolescence: A Public Health Concern
Hatim A Omar, Donald E Greydanus, Dilip R Patel and Joav Merrick (Editors)
2009. ISBN: 978-1-60692-821-9

Poverty and Children: A Public Health Concern
Alexis Lieberman and Joav Merrick (Editors)
2009. ISBN: 978-1-60741-140-6

Living on the Edge: The Mythical, Spiritual, and Philosophical Roots of Social Marginality
Joseph Goodbread
2009. ISBN: 978-1-60741-162-8 (Hardcover)
2011. ISBN: 978-1-61470-192-7 (E-book)
2013. ISBN: 978-1-61122-986-8 (Softcover)

Social and Cultural Psychiatry Experience from the Caribbean Region
Hari D Maharajh and Joav Merrick (Editors)
2011. ISBN: 978-1-61668-506-5

Challenges in Adolescent Health: An Australian Perspective
David Bennett, Susan Towns and Elizabeth Elliott and Joav Merrick (Editors)
2009. ISBN: 978-1-60741-616-6

Children and Pain
P Schofield and J Merrick (Editors)
2009. ISBN: 978-1-60876-020-6

Alcohol-Related Cognitive Disorders: Research and Clinical Perspectives
Leo Sher, Isack Kandel and Joav Merrick (Editors)
2009. ISBN: 978-1-60741-730-9

Bone and Brain Metastases: Advances in Research and Treatment
Arjun Sahgal, Edward Chow and Joav Merrick (Editors)
2010. ISBN: 978-1-61668-365-8

Chance Action and Therapy: The Playful Way of Changing
Uri Wernik
2010. ISBN: 978-1-60876-393-1

International Aspects of Child Abuse and Neglect
Howard Dubowitz and Joav Merrick (Editors)
2010. ISBN: 978-1-61122-049-0

Behavioral Pediatrics, 3rd Edition
Donald E Greydanus, Dilip R Patel, Helen D Pratt and Joseph L Calles Jr. (Editors)
2011. ISBN: 978-1-60692-702-1

Advances in Environmental Health Effects of Toxigenic Mold and Mycotoxins
Ebere Cyril Anyanwu
2011. ISBN: 978-1-60741-953-2

Rural Child Health: International Aspects
Erica Bell and Joav Merrick (Editors)
2011. ISBN: 978-1-60876-357-3

Principles of Holistic Psychiatry: A Textbook on Holistic Medicine for Mental Disorders
Soren Ventegodt and Joav Merrick
2011. ISBN: 978-1-61761-940-3

International Aspects of Child Abuse and Neglect
Howard Dubowitz and Joav Merrick (Editors)
2011. ISBN: 978-1-60876-703-8

Positive Youth Development: Evaluation and Future Directions in a Chinese Context
Daniel TL Shek, Hing Keung Ma and Joav Merrick (Editors)
2011. ISBN: 978-1-60876-830-1

Alternative Medicine Yearbook 2009
Joav Merrick (Editor)
2011. ISBN: 978-1-61668-910-0

Understanding Eating Disorders: Integrating Culture, Psychology and Biology
Yael Latzer, Joav Merrick and Daniel Stein (Editors)
2011. ISBN: 978-1-61728-298-0

Advanced Cancer, Pain and Quality of Life
Edward Chow and Joav Merrick (Editors)
2011. ISBN: 978-1-61668-207-1

Positive Youth Development: Implementation of a Youth Program in a Chinese Context
Daniel TL Shek, Hing Keung Ma and Joav Merrick (Editors)
2011. ISBN: 978-1-61668-230-9

Environment, Mood Disorders and Suicide
Teodor T Postolache and Joav Merrick (Editors)
2011. ISBN: 978-1-61668-505-8

Chance Action and Therapy: The Playful Way of Changing
Uri Wernik
2011. ISBN: 978-1-61122-987-5

Public Health Yearbook 2009
Joav Merrick (Editor)
2011. ISBN: 978-1-61668-911-7

Child Health and Human Development Yearbook 2009
Joav Merrick (Editor)
2011. ISBN: 978-1-61668-912-4

Narratives and Meanings of Migration
Julia Mirsky
2011. ISBN: 978-1-61761-103-2

Self-Management and the Health Care Consumer
Peter William Harvey
2011. ISBN: 978-1-61761-796-6

Sexology from a Holistic Point of View
Soren Ventegodt and Joav Merrick
2011. ISBN: 978-1-61761-859-8

Clinical Aspects of Psychopharmacology in Childhood and Adolescence
DE Greydanus, JL Calles Jr., DP Patel, A Nazeer and J Merrick (Editors)
2011. ISBN: 978-1-61122-135-0

**Drug Abuse in Hong Kong:
Development and Evaluation of
a Prevention Program**
*Daniel TL Shek, Rachel CF Sun
and Joav Merrick (Editors)*
2011. ISBN: 978-1-61324-491-3

Climate Change and Rural Child Health
*Erica Bell, Bastian M Seidel
and Joav Merrick (Editors)*
2011. ISBN: 978-1-61122-640-9

**Rural Medical Education:
Practical Strategies**
*Erica Bell and Craig Zimitat
and Joav Merrick (Editors)*
2011. ISBN: 978-1-61122-649-2

**Understanding Eating Disorders:
Integrating Culture,
Psychology and Biology**
*Yael Latzer, Joav Merrick
and Daniel Stein (Editors)*
2011. ISBN: 978-1-61470-976-3

**Positive Youth Development: Evaluation
and Future Directions
in a Chinese Context**
*Daniel TL Shek, Hing Keung Ma and Joav
Merrick (Editors)*
2011. ISBN: 978-1-62100-175-1

**The Dance of Sleeping and Eating
among Adolescents: Normal and
Pathological Perspectives**
Yael Latzer and Orna Tzischinsky (Editors)
2011. ISBN: 978-1-61209-710-7

**Randomized Clinical Trials and
Placebo: Can You Trust the Drugs Are
Working and Safe?**
Søren Ventegodt and Joav Merrick
2011. ISBN: 978-1-61470-151-4 (E-book)
2012. ISBN: 978-1-61470-067-8 (Hardcover)

**Child and Adolescent
Health Yearbook 2009**
Joav Merrick (Editor)
2012. ISBN: 978-1-61668-913-1

**Applied Public Health: Examining
Multifaceted Social or Ecological
Problems and Child Maltreatment**
John R Lutzker and Joav Merrick (Editors)
2012. ISBN: 978-1-62081-356-0

**Adolescence and Chronic Illness.
A Public Health Concern**
*Hatim Omar, Donald E Greydanus,
Dilip R Patel and Joav Merrick (Editors)*
2012. ISBN: 978-1-60876-628-4

**Translational Research for
Primary Healthcare**
*Erica Bell, Gert P Westert
and Joav Merrick (Editors)*
2012. ISBN: 978-1-61324-647-4

**Child and Adolescent Health
Yearbook 2010**
Joav Merrick (Editor)
2012. ISBN: 978-1-61209-788-6

**Child Health and Human Development
Yearbook 2010**
Joav Merrick (Editor)
2012. ISBN: 8-1-61209-789-3

Public Health Yearbook 2010
Joav Merrick (Editor)
2012. ISBN: 978-1-61209-971-2

**The Astonishing Brain and Holistic
Consciousness: Neuroscience
and Vedanta Perspectives**
Vinod D Deshmukh
2012. ISBN: 978-1-61324-295-7

**Treatment and Recovery
of Eating Disorders**
Daniel Stein and Yael Latzer (Editors)
2012. ISBN: 978-1-61470-259-7 (Hardcover)
2013. ISBN: 978-1-62808-248-7 (Softcover)

Alternative Medicine Yearbook 2010
Joav Merrick (Editor)
2012. ISBN: 978-1-62100-132-4

**Building Community Capacity:
Minority and Immigrant Populations**
*Rosemary M Caron and
Joav Merrick (Editors)*
2012. ISBN: 978-1-62081-022-4

**Human Immunodeficiency Virus (HIV)
Research: Social Science Aspects**
Hugh Klein and Joav Merrick (Editors)
2012. ISBN: 978-1-62081-293-8

**AIDS and Tuberculosis:
Public Health Aspects**
Daniel Chemtob and Joav Merrick (Editors)
2012. ISBN: 978-1-62081-382-9

Public Health Yearbook 2011
Joav Merrick (Editor)
2012. ISBN: 978-1-62081-433-8

**Alternative Medicine Research
Yearbook 2011**
Joav Merrick (Editor)
2012. ISBN: 978-1-62081-476-5

**Textbook on Evidence-Based Holistic
Mind-Body Medicine: Basic Principles
of Healing in Traditional
Hippocratic Medicine**
Søren Ventegodt and Joav Merrick
2012. ISBN: 978-1-62257-094-2

**Textbook on Evidence-Based Holistic
Mind-Body Medicine: Holistic Practice
of Traditional Hippocratic Medicine**
Søren Ventegodt and Joav Merrick
2012. ISBN: 978-1-62257-105-5

**Textbook on Evidence-Based Holistic
Mind-Body Medicine: Healing the Mind
in Traditional Hippocratic Medicine**
Søren Ventegodt and Joav Merrick
2012. ISBN: 978-1-62257-112-3

**Textbook on Evidence-Based Holistic
Mind-Body Medicine: Sexology and
Traditional Hippocratic Medicine**
Søren Ventegodt and Joav Merrick
2012. ISBN: 978-1-62257-130-7

**Textbook on Evidence-Based Holistic
Mind-Body Medicine: Research,
Philosophy, Economy and Politics of
Traditional Hippocratic Medicine**
Søren Ventegodt and Joav Merrick
2012. ISBN: 978-1-62257-140-6

**Building Community Capacity:
Skills and Principles**
*Rosemary M Caron and Joav Merrick
(Editors)*
2012. ISBN 978-1-61209-331-4

**Our Search for Meaning in Life:
Quality of Life Philosophy**
Soren Ventegodt and Joav Merrick
2012. ISBN: 978-1-61470-494-2

**Health and Happiness from Meaningful
Work: Research in Quality
of Working Life**
*Soren Ventegodt and Joav Merrick
(Editors)*
2013. ISBN: 978-1-60692-820-2

Pediatric and Adolescent Sexuality and Gynecology: Principles for the Primary Care Clinician
Hatim A Omar, Donald E Greydanus,
Artemis K Tsitsika, Dilip R Patel
and Joav Merrick (Editors)
2013. ISBN: 978-1-60876-735-9

Conceptualizing Behavior in Health and Social Research: A Practical Guide to Data Analysis
Said Shahtahmasebi and Damon Berridge
2013. ISBN: 978-1-60876-383-2

Adolescence and Sports
Dilip R Patel, Donald E Greydanus,
Hatim Omar and Joav Merrick (Editors)
2013. ISBN: 978-1-60876-702-1

Human Development: Biology from a Holistic Point of View
Søren Ventegodt, Tyge Dahl Hermansen
and Joav Merrick (Editors)
2013. ISBN: 978-1-61470-441-6

Building Community Capacity: Case Examples from Around the World
Rosemary M Caron
and Joav Merrick (Editors)
2013. ISBN: 978-1-62417-175-8

Managed Care in a Public Setting
Richard Evan Steele
2013. ISBN: 978-1-62417-970-9

Alternative Medicine Research Yearbook 2012
Søren Ventegodt and Joav Merrick (Editors)
2013. ISBN: 978-1-62808-080-3

Health Promotion: Community Singing as a Vehicle to Promote Health
Joav Merrick (Editors)
2013. ISBN: 978-1-62618-908-9

Public Health Yearbook 2012
Joav Merrick (Editor)
2013. ISBN: 978-1-62808-078-0

Health Risk Communication
Marijke Lemal and Joav Merrick (Editors)
2013. ISBN: 978-1-62257-544-2

Bullying: A Public Health Concern
Jorge C Srabstein
and Joav Merrick (Editors)
2013. ISBN: 978-1-62618-564-7

Advanced Cancer: Managing Symptoms and Quality of Life
Natalie Pulenzas, Breanne Lechner,
Nemica Thavarajah, Edward Chow
and Joav Merrick (Editors)
2013. ISBN: 978-1-62808-239-5

Health Promotion: Strengthening Positive Health and Preventing Disease
Jing Sun, Nicholas Buys
and Joav Merrick (Editors)
2013. ISBN: 978-1-62257-870-2

Pain Management Yearbook 2011
Joav Merrick (Editor)
2013. ISBN: 978-1-62808-970-7

Pain Management Yearbook 2012
Joav Merrick (Editor)
2013. ISBN: 978-1-62808-973-8

Food, Nutrition and Eating Behavior
Joav Merrick and Sigal Israeli
2013. ISBN: 978-1-62948-233-0

Public Health Concern: Smoking, Alcohol and Substance Use
Joav Merrick
and Ariel Tenenbaum (Editors)
2013. ISBN: 978-1-62948-424-2

Mental Health from an International Perspective
Joav Merrick, Shoshana Aspler and Mohammed Morad (Editors)
2013. ISBN: 978-1-62948-519-5

Suicide from a Public Health Perspective
Said Shahtahmasebi and Joav Merrick
2014. ISBN: 978-1-62948-536-2

India: Health and Human Development Aspects
Joav Merrick (Editor)
2014. ISBN: 978-1-62948-784-7

Alternative Medicine Research Yearbook 2013
Joav Merrick (Editor)
2014. ISBN: 978-1-63321-094-3

Public Health Yearbook 2013
Joav Merrick (Editor)
2014. ISBN: 978-1-63321-095-0

Public Health: Improving Health via Inter-Professional Collaborations
Rosemary M. Caron and Joav Merrick (Editors)
2014. ISBN: 978-1-63321-569-6

Pain Management Yearbook 2014
Joav Merrick (Editor)
2015. ISBN: 978-1-63482-164-3

Public Health Yearbook 2014
Joav Merrick (Editor)
2015. ISBN: 978-1-63482-165-0

Forensic Psychiatry: A Public Health Perspective
Leo Sher and Joav Merrick (Editors)
2015. ISBN: 978-1-63483-339-4

Leadership and Service Learning Education: Holistic Development for Chinese University Students
Daniel TL Shek, Florence KY Wu and Joav Merrick (Editors)
2015. ISBN: 978-1-63483-340-0

HEALTH AND HUMAN DEVELOPMENT

MENTAL AND HOLISTIC HEALTH

SOME INTERNATIONAL PERSPECTIVES

**JOSEPH L. CALLES JR.
DONALD E. GREYDANUS
AND
JOAV MERRICK
EDITORS**

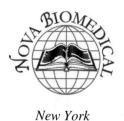

New York

Copyright © 2015 by Nova Science Publishers, Inc.

All rights reserved. No part of this book may be reproduced, stored in a retrieval system or transmitted in any form or by any means: electronic, electrostatic, magnetic, tape, mechanical photocopying, recording or otherwise without the written permission of the Publisher.

We have partnered with Copyright Clearance Center to make it easy for you to obtain permissions to reuse content from this publication. Simply navigate to this publication's page on Nova's website and locate the "Get Permission" button below the title description. This button is linked directly to the title's permission page on copyright.com. Alternatively, you can visit copyright.com and search by title, ISBN, or ISSN.

For further questions about using the service on copyright.com, please contact:
Copyright Clearance Center
Phone: +1-(978) 750-8400   Fax: +1-(978) 750-4470   E-mail: info@copyright.com.

NOTICE TO THE READER
The Publisher has taken reasonable care in the preparation of this book, but makes no expressed or implied warranty of any kind and assumes no responsibility for any errors or omissions. No liability is assumed for incidental or consequential damages in connection with or arising out of information contained in this book. The Publisher shall not be liable for any special, consequential, or exemplary damages resulting, in whole or in part, from the readers' use of, or reliance upon, this material. Any parts of this book based on government reports are so indicated and copyright is claimed for those parts to the extent applicable to compilations of such works.

Independent verification should be sought for any data, advice or recommendations contained in this book. In addition, no responsibility is assumed by the publisher for any injury and/or damage to persons or property arising from any methods, products, instructions, ideas or otherwise contained in this publication.

This publication is designed to provide accurate and authoritative information with regard to the subject matter covered herein. It is sold with the clear understanding that the Publisher is not engaged in rendering legal or any other professional services. If legal or any other expert assistance is required, the services of a competent person should be sought. FROM A DECLARATION OF PARTICIPANTS JOINTLY ADOPTED BY A COMMITTEE OF THE AMERICAN BAR ASSOCIATION AND A COMMITTEE OF PUBLISHERS.

Additional color graphics may be available in the e-book version of this book.

Library of Congress Cataloging-in-Publication Data

ISBN: 978-1-63483-589-3
Library of Congress Control Number: 2015947576

Published by Nova Science Publishers, Inc. † New York

CONTENTS

Introduction   1

Chapter 1   Introduction to mental and holistic health   3
Donald E Greydanus, Joseph L Calles Jr and Joav Merrick

Section one: Mental health issues   9

Chapter 2   Neuropsychiatric disorders: Attention deficit hyperactivity disorder   11
Joseph L Calles Jr.

Chapter 3   Neuropsychiatric disorders: Oppositional defiant and conduct disorders   29
Joseph L Calles Jr.

Chapter 4   Aggressive behaviors   41
Joseph L Calles Jr.

Chapter 5   Two depressive disorders: Major depressive and dysthymic disorders   59
Joseph L Calles Jr.

Chapter 6   Chronic illness: Pediatric bipolar disorder   75
Amy E West and Mani N Pavuluri

Chapter 7   Fear and anxiety disorders in children and adolescents   93
Lauren Boydston, William P French and Christopher K Varley

Chapter 8   Psychiatric disorders: Obsessive compulsive disorder   105
William P French, Lauren Boydston and Christopher K Varley

Section two: A holistic worldview   117

Chapter 9   World Health Organization model list of essential medicines   119
Søren Ventegod

Chapter 10   Alternative medicine (Non-Drug Medicine, CAM) versus pharmacological medicine   135
Søren Ventegodt

Chapter 11	Medical use of the hallucinogenic tea Ayahuasca in Peru *Søren Ventegodt and Pavlina Kordova*	**141**
Chapter 12	South Africa and Botswana: Traditional healing and ritualized cannibalism *Søren Ventegodt and Pavlina Kordova*	**163**
Section three: Acknowledgments		**169**
Chapter 13	About the editors	**171**
Chapter 14	About the Department of Pediatric and Adolescent Medicine, Western Michigan University Homer Stryker MD School of Medicine (WMED), Kalamazoo, Michigan USA	**173**
Chapter 15	About the National Institute of Child Health and Human Development in Israel	**175**
Chapter 16	About the book series "Health and Human Development"	**179**
Section four: Index		**183**
Index		**185**

INTRODUCTION

In: Mental and Holistic Health: Some International Perspectives ISBN: 978-1-63483-589-3
Editors: J. Calles Jr., D. Greydanus and J. Merrick © 2015 Nova Science Publishers, Inc.

Chapter 1

INTRODUCTION TO MENTAL AND HOLISTIC HEALTH

Donald E Greydanus[*], *MD, DrHC (Athens),*
Joseph L Calles Jr.[†], *and Joav Merrick*[‡],
MD, MMedSci, DMSc

[1]Professor and Founding Chair, Department of Pediatric and Adolescent Medicine, Western Michigan University Homer Stryker MD School of Medicine, Kalamazoo, Michigan, United States

[2]Professor, Department of Psychiatry, Western Michigan University Homer Stryker MD School of Medicine, Kalamazoo, Michigan, United States

[3]Professor, Medical Director, Health Services, Division for Intellectual and Developmental Disabilities, Ministry of Social Affairs and Social Services, Jerusalem, Israel

> The young physician starts life with 20 drugs for each disease, and the old physician ends life with one drug for 20 diseases
>
> Sir William Osler, MD (1849-1919)

The search for optimal medications to support health has been part of human history since early times (1). One concept that was learned early in the human civilization was that medications can be harmful as well as potentially beneficial. Witness the Genesis 3:6 account of Adam and Eve and their demise from eating the "forbidden" fruit.

Folklore and anecdotal information dominated human knowledge for more than 50,000 years until the work of the Chinese emperor, Shen-Nung (2737 BC), who became a pristine, official, and erudite classifier of medicinal herbs (2). One of the classic paintings of that ruler, called the "red" emperor, is of him holding the leaves of Ephedra ("machuang") confirming the idea that our first medications derived from herbals.

---

[*] E-mail: Donald.greydanus@med.wmich.edu.
[†] E-mail: joseph.calles@med.wmich.edu.
[‡] E-mail: jmerrick@zahav.net.il.

Anecdotal evidence gained over thousands of years of the Chinese and Indian civilizations still remains essentially lost in Western civilization that slowly developed its own ideas of the best medications for medical and mental health. One of the earliest sources of a Western pharmacopoeia is from Egypt whose early scholars produced the 1550 BC Ebers Paprus, a classic scroll with 110 pages containing 700 formulas of vegetable, mineral, and animal origins (3).

The ancient Greek civilization began to develop principles of science though this did not benefit the search for pharmacologic agents until much later in the history of Western civilization. Athletes of the Ancient Olympics (776 BC to 393 AD) consumed various products in efforts to acquire optimal health and sports performance; these products included figs, mushrooms, strychnine, and others. While progress in some branches of science and philosophy were impressive in ancient Greece, discoveries in use of medicines to cure human malady was slow. Consider the lament of Aristotle, one of the most famous and brilliant of Greek philosophers, about the state of medicine in ancient Greece: "….the physician does not cure man, except in an incidental sense (4)." Indeed, clinical pharmacology had a long way to go!

A major reason for the slow progress of science in this regard was the reliance of human beings for thousands of years on conflicting dogmas based on a complex mix of mantics, haruspex, magic, and religion. This was the reaction of humans to a mystifying, cruel, and often violent world. Hippocrates of Cos (460 to 377 BC), the founder of medicine in Western civilization, began to turn this page with his Hippocraticum Corpus and his now classic dictum to observe one's patient.

Diseases were often blurred with attempts to understand magic and religion. Epilepsy and mental illness, for example, were blamed on demon possession and the treatment was exorcism, not pharmacological prescriptions. Claudius Galen (130-210 AD), the famous Greek physician and surgeon caring for the upper class of ancient Rome and its superstar gladiators, linked many diseases (including epilepsy and mental illness) to masturbation of adolescent and young adults. His concern with hebetic sexuality lingers with us even in the 21st century:

> Watch carefully over this young man, leave him alone neither day nor night; at least sleep in his chamber. When he has contracted this fatal habit (i.e., masturbation), the most fatal to which a young man can be subject, he will carry its painful effects to the tomb - his mind and body will always be enervated (5).

The fall of the Roman Empire in the 5th century AD led to a dramatic decline in scientific information as humans turned ever most desperately to magic, mysticism, and religion to deal with a violent and unforgiving environment. There were some bright spots that continued a flame of knowledge, such as the Persian physician Rhazes (Muhammad ibn Zakariya Razi; 865-925 AD) whose book on disorders of children began a serious look at this age group.

The West very gradually arose from it sycophantic and saturnine slumber. For example, a book that was released in the late 11th century that dealt with medical disorders of children called De Mylierum Passionibus by Trotula Platearius of Salerno, Italy. The development of the Renaissance (14th to 17th century in Europe) allowed an explosion of medical knowledge in areas of anatomy, physiology, surgery, and other areas (i.e., philosophy, art, language, others). Thomas Phaer (1510-1560) was a lawyer and physician in England who published the first book (The Boke of Chyldren) that made the first real distinction between the phase of childhood and that of adulthood.

As each century passed, more progress in understanding the causes of diseases occurred that allowed improvement in their management. Epidemics of major infections ravaged Europe, such as the Black plague due to Yersinia pestis leading to the death of one-third of those in Europe in the mid-14th century. Dr. Edward Jenner (1749-1823) was a general physician in England whose landmark observations and experimentation with cowpox in the latter part of the 18th century led to smallpox vaccine development and eventually the tremendous triumphs of vaccinology in the 20th and 21st centuries (6).

The term "biology" was launched in the early 19th century and initiated the attempts to separate out etiology of diseases from ancient and persistent philosophical theories (1). Old theories of anatomy were challenged by Andreas Versalius (1514-1564) in Italy with his classic De Humani Corporis. Concepts of blood circulation were provided a modern view by William Harvey in England based on earlier work such as that of the Arabic physician, Ibn al-Nafic (1242), the father of circulatory physiology. The theories of Hippocrates and Galen were finally challenged amidst a stunning milieu of intellectual curiosity and inquiry. A pathologist in Ohio, USA, Dr. John Scudder, wrote a pediatric textbook challenging the notion that treatment of adults would suffice for children. He noted: "there are sufficient differences in the action of remedies upon the adult and child, to demand a careful study of the subject" (i.e., the child) (7).

The seeds of pharmacology were set by the Red Emperor, Shen-Nung (2737 BC) and the Egyptian Ebers Paprus (1550 BC). Pedanius Dioscorides (40 to 90 AD) was a surgeon and botanist in Rome whose travels around the Roman Empire led to his classic work on herbal and medicinal products, De Materia Medica (Regarding Medical Matters (8, 9). This pharmacopeia influenced medical treatment for over a millennium. The Persian physician and chemist, Avicenna (Ibn Sina) (980-1037 AD) wrote a medical textbook, The Canon of Medicine, that became a standard of pharmacologic regimens for the next 6 centuries.

After thousands of years of observations, the modern era of clinical pharmacology can be traced to the English physician, William Withering (1741-1799); he was also a chemist and botanist who discovered digitalis (Foxglove) and carefully wrote about both its benefits for heart failure and also its toxic effects. The first department of pharmacology was developed by Rudolf Buchheim (1820-1879) at the University of Giessen, Germany in 1847.

The marching progress of the 17th and 18th centuries led to an explosion of new knowledge in various fields of science in the 20th centuries. Work in clinical pharmacology escalated in new drugs for medicine and psychiatry in children, adolescents, and adults. Though Hippocrates recommended willow-leaf tea (containing salicylates) for relief of pain and fever, it was not until 1897 that chemists Felix Hoffmann and Arthur Eichengrün identified acetylsalicylic acid which was then marketed in 1899 as Aspirin (10). Canadian surgeon Frederick Banting and medical student Charles Best identified insulin in 1922 which became the drug prolonging the lives of countless numbers of people with diabetes mellitus in the 20th and 21st centuries (11). Sir Alexander Fleming, a Scottish biologist and pharmacologist, identified penicillin from mold (Penicillium notatum) in 1928 stimulating the further development of antibiotics.

Pharmacology had arrived after thousands of years of observation with more and more drugs identified as being beneficial. Psychiatrist Charles Bradley published his landmark study in 1937 observing the benefit of a stimulant Benzedrine (racemic mixture of dextroamphetamine and levoamphetamine) on 30 children with various mental health conditions including what would later be called attention deficit hyperactivity disorder (ADHD) (12). In the same year researchers Molitich and Eccles published one of the first placebo-control research studies on the benefit of Benzedrine on 93 youths labeled as juvenile delinquents (13).

Edward Kendall was an American chemist at the Mayo Clinic (Rochester, Minnesota, USA) who identified cortisone in 1949 along with the help of others, such as physician Philip Hench (14). Chlorpromazine was introduced in 1950 as the beginning of antipsychotic medication that has now evolved into the second and third generation of antipsychotics (15, 16). The Argentine child psychiatrist, M. Knobel, identified the stimulant, methylphenidate, as beneficial for children with ADHD, and then called hyperkinesis with organicity (17). In the 1950s famous sex educator Margaret Sanger, researcher Gregory Pincus, and physician John Rock became protagonists in the incredible story that lead to the development of Enovid which became an FDA-approved drug for menstrual disorders in 1957 and FDA-approved oral contraceptive in 1960 (18).

Ace inhibitors were introduced in 1956 based on the work of Leonard Skegg and ibuprofen was introduced in 1969 based on the work of chemist John Nicholson and pharmacologist Stewart Adams from Nottingham, England (19).

Research has continued and each decade has produced more and more drugs for the benefit of medical and mental health (20). However, pharmacologic trials are increasingly directed more by the pharmaceutical industry than independent researchers, raising concerns over the validity and neutrality of such research (16, 21, 22). It must be remembered that each drug has side effects and the risk of benefit to adverse profile must be carefully identified in a neutral and non-biased manner for the benefit of the patient (23). It is important to note that the word pharmacology comes from the Greek work, pharmakon, with the dual meaning of "poison" in classic Greek and "drugs" in Modern Greek. Some drugs can be poison and clinicians must monitor both positive and negative aspects of drug administration very carefully and obsessively. Plants can be wondrous, as noted with willow leaf (salicylates) or foxglove (Digitalis purpurea) but also deceptively dangerous as seen with Cannabis sativa (marijuana) or Erythroxylon coca (cocaine).

Pharmacologic management of human disease is clearly part of the 21st century medical armamentarium. Adolescents of this second decade of the 21st century and those adolescents soon to come will determine the outcome of our planet and life into the 22nd century. Pharmacology will remain an ever-growing part of clinician's efforts to improve their patients' mental and medical health.

REFERENCES

[1] Magner LN. A history of the life sciences, 3rd Edition. New York: Marcel Dekker, 2002.
[2] Greydanus DE, Patel DR. Sports doping in athletes. Pediatr Clin North Am 2010;57(3):729-50.
[3] Scholl R. Der Papyrus Ebers. Die grösste Buchrolle zur Heilkunde Altägyptens. Leipzig, Germany: Schriften aus der Universitätsbibliothek 7, 2002. [German]
[4] Wheelwright P. Aristotle. New York: Odyssey Press, 1951:68.
[5] Greydanus DE, Geller B. Masturbation: historical perspective. NY State Med 1980;80:1892-6.

[6] Koppaka R. Ten great public health achievements—United States, 2001-2010. MMWR 2011;60(19):619-23.
[7] Scudder NJM. The eclectic practice of diseases of children, Cincinnati, OH: American Publishing Co, 1869:19.
[8] Brater DC, Daly WJ. Clinical pharmacology in the Middle Ages: principles that presage the 21st century." Clin Pharmacol Ther 2000; 67(5):447–50.
[9] Vallance P, Smart TG. The future of pharmacology. Br J Pharmacol.
[10] 2006;147(Suppl 1):S304–7.
[11] Griffiths R. The discovery of aspirin. Am Philatelist 2003;34:701-7.
[12] Hughes E. Breakthrough: The discovery of insulin and the making of a medical miracle. New York: St Martin Press, 2010.
[13] Bradley C. The behavior of children receiving Benzedrine. Am J Psychiatry 1937;94:577-85.
[14] Molitch M, Eccles AK. The effect of Benzedrine sulfate on the intelligence scores of children. Am J Psychiatry 1937;94:577-85.
[15] Woodward RB, Sondheimer F, Taub D. The total synthesis of cortisone. J Am Chem Soc 1951;73:4057.
[16] Greydanus DE, Patel DR, Feucht D. Preface: Pediatric and adolescent psychopharmacology: The past, the present, and the future. Pediatr Clin North Am 2011; 58(1): xv-xxiv.
[17] López-Munoz F, Alamo C, Cuenca E, Shen WW, Clervoy P, Rubio G. History and discover and clinical introduction of chlorpromazine. Ann Clin Psychiatry 2005; 17(3):113-35.
[18] Knobel M, Wolman M, Mason A. Hyperkinesis and organicity in children. Arch Gen Psychiatry 1959;1(3):310-21.
[19] Bynum WF. The western medical tradition. Cambridge, England: Cambridge University Press, 2006.
[20] Moore N. Forty years of ibuprofen use. Int J Clin Pract 2003; 135:28-31.
[21] Greydanus DE, Calles Jr JL, Patel DR. Pediatric and adolescent psychopharmacology. Cambridge, England: Cambridge University Press, 2008.
[22] Greydanus DE, Patel DR. The role of pharmaceutical influence in education and research: The clinician's response. Asian J Paediatr Pract 2006;9: 35-41.
[23] Kölch M, Ludolph AG, Plener PL, Fangerau H, Vitiello B, Fegert JM. Safeguarding children's rights in psychopharmacological research: Ethical and legal issues. Curr Pharm Des 2010; 16(22):2398-406.
[24] Ventegodt S, Greydanus DE, Merrick J. Alternative medicine does not exist, biomedicine does not exist, there is only evidence–based medicine. Int J Adolesc Med 2011;23(3):7-10.

Section one: Mental health issues

In: Mental and Holistic Health: Some International Perspectives ISBN: 978-1-63483-589-3
Editors: J. Calles Jr., D. Greydanus and J. Merrick © 2015 Nova Science Publishers, Inc.

Chapter 2

NEUROPSYCHIATRIC DISORDERS: ATTENTION DEFICIT HYPERACTIVITY DISORDER

Joseph L Calles Jr.[*], *MD*

Department of Psychiatry, Western Michigan University Homer Stryker MD School of Medicine, Kalamazoo, Michigan, United States

Attention deficit hyperactivity disorder (ADHD) is a common neuropsychiatric disorder that is routinely encountered in general pediatric practice. However, it remains underdiagnosed and undertreated. The potential long-term, negative sequelae of ADHD include academic and occupational underachievement, unstable interpersonal relationships, substance abuse, and legal difficulties. This paper will review ADHD's clinical characteristics, diagnostic criteria, common comorbid conditions, and therapeutic interventions, including selected non-pharmacologic treatments.

INTRODUCTION

Attention deficit hyperactivity disorder (ADHD) is a neurobehavioral disorder that is fairly common in the general population and even more commonly seen in clinical practice. It tends to be highly variable in terms of symptomatic presentation, degree of functional impairment, comorbidity, and persistence into adulthood. Despite its common nature, ADHD can still be problematic to pediatricians in terms of its assessment, and even more so its treatment.

---

[*] Correspondence: Professor Joseph L Calles Jr, Department of Psychiatry, Western Michigan University Homer Stryker MD School of Medicine, 1717 Shaffer Road, Suite 010, Kalamazoo, MI 49048, United States. E-mail: joseph.calles@med.wmich.edu.

DEFINITION

The core symptoms of ADHD are currently divided into two categories: 1) *inattention* and 2) *hyperactivity-impulsivity*. These features are commonly seen in many children and adolescents, so in order to differentiate the clinical disorder from more normal behaviors, symptoms must be present for *at least 6 months*; in addition, the following conditions must be met: 1) symptoms must be *maladaptive*, i.e., must impair functioning vs. just being bothersome; 2) symptoms must be *developmentally inappropriate*, i.e., would be consistent with a much younger age; 3) several symptoms must be present, to a significant degree, *before the age of 12 years* (1,2); 4) symptoms are *displayed in more than one setting*, i.e., not just at school or just at home; and 5) the symptom complex *does not co-occur exclusively* with another disorder, nor is it *better accounted for* by other disorders (e.g., psychotic, mood, anxiety, dissociative, or personality disorders).

Table 1. DSM-5 ADHD subtypes and associated symptoms

Combined (ADHD-C)	• ≥6* symptoms of inattention • ≥6* symptoms of hyperactivity-impulsivity • Both have been present for at least 6 months
Predominantly Inattentive (ADHD-I)	• ≥ 6* symptoms of inattention present for at least 6 months • <6* symptoms of hyperactivity-impulsivity or symptoms have not been present for at least 6 months
Predominantly Hyperactive-Impulsive (ADHD-H)	• ≥6* symptoms of hyperactivity-impulsivity present for at least 6 months • <6* symptoms of inattention or symptoms have not been present for at least 6 months

* Out of a total of 9 possible symptoms in each of the two clusters.

In the new "Diagnostic and statistical manual of mental disorders, Fifth Edition (DSM-5)" (3), there are three presentations (types) of ADHD: Combined (ADHD-C), Predominantly Inattentive (ADHD-I), and Predominantly Hyperactive-Impulsive (ADHD-H). Table 1 describes the features of each ADHD subtype.

EPIDEMIOLOGY

The prevalence rates reported for ADHD vary greatly around the world (4). There are several factors that seem to account for the variability: 1) Diagnostic criteria utilized, e.g., the prevalence of ADHD is higher in newer studies that used DSM-IV vs. older studies that used DSM-III or DSM-III-R; 2) Sources of information, i.e., teachers report higher rates of ADHD symptoms than do parents; 3) Impairment status, e.g., prevalence rates of ADHD are higher when functional impairment is excluded as a diagnostic criterion and 4) Geographic location, e.g., there is greater congruence between American and European studies vs. greater incongruence between American studies and those from developing countries. Taking all of these issues into consideration, the overall prevalence world-wide of ADHD has been calculated as 5.29% (5).

Prevalence rates of ADHD also vary based on individual characteristics. For example, studies have consistently shown that the ratio of boys-to-girls with ADHD is about 2:1. In clinical settings ADHD-C is the most commonly encountered type, whereas in community studies ADHD-I is the most common type (representing about one-half of the ADHD sample). The ADHD-H type is primarily seen in the preschool age group, with steady declines into adolescence; conversely, the ADHD-I type is uncommon in preschoolers, very common in adolescents.

There are inconsistent findings regarding age at first diagnosis of ADHD, but affected younger children seem to be more readily recognized, especially when they begin school. However, it has been shown that the relative age of a student (i.e., where the child's birthday falls relative to the cutoff date for starting school) has a significant effect on teachers' perceptions of the presence of ADHD symptoms. In other words, the younger the child is (compared to same-grade classmates), the more likely that he or she will be diagnosed with ADHD. Finally, the true prevalence of ADHD in children from minority and under-represented groups is difficult to gauge, in that the parents of those children tend to deny, minimize or normalize ADHD-like behaviors, whereas the teachers of those children tend to over-report symptoms (6).

CLINICAL FEATURES

The types and ratios of ADHD symptoms not uncommonly change over time (7), and depend to some extent on the child's developmental level. The following clinical ADHD descriptions are divided into four broad age categories: preschoolers (3-5½ years); school-age (6-12 years); adolescents (13-18 years); and, college-age young adults (18-22 years).

ADHD in preschoolers (8). The parents of young children with ADHD usually report a long history of fairly dramatic symptoms. Hyperactivity and impulsivity dominate the clinical picture. Excessive activity is expressed motorically, and the children are described as if they have a "motor running" inside of them, are in motion "non-stop" and "can't sit still," or "wear everyone out," including other children. Verbal activity is also excessive, and the children may be called "chatterboxes" or "motormouths," and may ask questions incessantly, even about things that they already know the answers to. They find it difficult to stay in their seats beyond brief periods of time, and family members may report that the children eat while standing up or walking in place at the table (in extreme cases the parents may follow the children around and put the food into their mouths!). In the daycare or preschool setting young children with ADHD exhibit similar motor and verbal activities. They often cannot participate in calmer indoor activities, such as coloring or putting puzzles together. They may have trouble settling down during rest periods, and many will not take a nap. They may monopolize classroom discussions or interfere with stories being read by the teacher. Even outdoor play may be problematic, as the children tend to be excitable, aggressive and difficult to re-direct.

If the hyperactivity weren't enough for the caring adults to deal with, young ADHD children also demonstrate impulsivity, i.e., the spontaneous motor or verbal actions that are expressed without regard for their appropriateness or their potential for being disruptive- or even dangerous. These children have been known to climb to high places, find themselves in precarious situations (e.g., being trapped), or run into traffic, all without regard to their own safety. They are careless in their play, such that injuries are more common in young children with ADHD vs. in those without it. The injuries themselves are not the routine "bumps and bruises" of childhood. Lacerations that require suturing, long bone fractures, concussions, burns, and ingestions of toxic substances are over-represented in this group of children.

All young children have relatively short attention spans (minutes at a time) (9), but those with ADHD may only be able to sustain focus for seconds. Their interest in things also lasts only briefly, and they seem to require near-constant attention and stimulation. The combination of hyperactivity, impulsivity and inattention alienates peers and "burns out" caregivers. In addition, the associated low frustration tolerance, irritability and tendency towards aggression make it difficult for parents to take the children into public settings. They may tantrum in stores, become disruptive in restaurants, and may be "kicked out" of daycare and preschool. If the parents themselves share similar characteristics (or even have ADHD), their level of frustration and anger could rise to the point that physical punishments are used, placing the children at risk of being physically abused.

Biological rhythms may also be disturbed. Sleep onset may be delayed for up to hours and there may be frequent awakenings during the night; sometimes the children will not fall back asleep. Despite the low quantity of sleep, ADHD children may still awaken very early in the morning. The parents' sleep will also be disrupted, as they will get up to monitor the children and try to prevent injuries or other damages (such as playing with the stove and starting a fire). Appetite can be quite variable. Some ADHD children are picky and may eat only enough to briefly eliminate hunger pains; other children may eat large amounts of food, even to the point of feeling sick. There may be delays in attaining bladder control, and bedwetting may occur.

ADHD in school-age children

As ADHD children transition into elementary education their inattentive symptoms become more pronounced. Studies in this age group consistently show that one-half of all ADHD children meet criteria for ADHD-I. However, the diagnosis can be missed if the inattention is not accompanied by obvious hyperactivity or impulsivity, as the cognitive symptoms may be relatively subtle when compared to the motor and verbal symptoms. It is the poor attention span and easy distractibility that contributes to the poor academic functioning seen in most ADHD children. Disorganization is often a related feature. These children tend to "lose" things, such as classroom assignments, textbooks, pencils and other supplies, money, articles of clothing, etc. Their personal areas- desks, bins, lockers, etc. - are like "black holes," i.e., everything goes into them and nothing seems to come out again.

When hyperactivity and/or impulsivity are prominent, as in ADHD-H or ADHD-C, the children display disruptive behaviors, such as talking to peers during work periods, getting out of their seats without permission (frequently visiting the pencil sharpener seems to be a favorite), and blurting out answers to questions without raising their hands. In more extreme cases children may fall out of their seats, crawl around on the floor or under their desks, physically touch classmates or their belongings, or engage in play activities when they are supposed to be working. They find it difficult- or even impossible- to read quietly to themselves or to work independently. Children may be forced to sit close to teachers in order to be redirected more readily. Sometimes children are isolated away from peers in an attempt to reduce environmental stimulation; this may be in a back corner of the classroom, or even outside in the hallway. When classroom management strategies fail, ADHD children may be sent to the office. A persistent pattern of losing classroom time may prompt a referral to a smaller, self-contained classroom setting.

In addition to formal academic learning, schools also provides the opportunity for social learning. ADHD children also struggle in the social realm. There is a correlation between hyperactive/impulsive symptoms and being disliked by peers, which in turn may be related to socially inappropriate behaviors. ADHD children can be very impatient, and may alienate other children by not being able to wait their turns or follow the rules during games.

The behaviors demonstrated at school are mirrored at home. Family routines may be disrupted by the children's ADHD symptoms. Parents describe nighttimes and mornings as being especially problematic. At night the children may have difficulty settling down (e.g., stopping play) and getting ready for bed, leading to "battles." In the morning there may be struggles in getting the children out of bed, and once up they may need frequent reminders or even assistance in getting ready for school (e.g., the children who are supposed to be brushing their teeth may be found watching TV). An especially common area of conflict centers on homework. ADHD children may not bring their books and assignments home, procrastinate in getting their work started, are easily distracted while working, may rush through their work (in order to get back to playing), and may not study for tests. Parents may have to sit with the children to keep them on task, and some parents may even do the work for the children to reduce their own time commitment and level of frustration. The issues related to homework may also be seen in chores, which can be "forgotten," sloppily rushed through, or even refused to be done by the children.

ADHD in adolescents

During adolescence there is a tendency for the hyperactivity and impulsivity of ADHD to attenuate (10). Despite that apparent change for the better, the majority of adolescents with ADHD will still meet the DSM-5 criteria for the disorder, will still have some functional impairment, and will still benefit from treatment. Although calmer in the classroom, these adolescents may continue to be inattentive, off-task, distractible, forgetful and disorganized. Grades may stay low or drop from previous levels. Interest in- and motivation for- school may be low, with associated poor academic effort. Faced with ongoing frustration and poor performance in the classroom, adolescents with ADHD may start skipping school, and are at high risk of dropping-out before graduating.

The adolescents with ADHD may fare no better at home. As they are now older but no more responsible than when younger, arguments with parents may increase and escalate even to the point of physical confrontations. The previously overactive children may now be sluggish and "lazy" teenagers, refusing to interact with their families and do their fair share of chores. Their mode of dress may become slovenly and personal hygiene may be neglected, most likely due to forgetfulness, but possibly secondary to comorbid psychiatric issues (see the next section on "Diagnosis"). This is the time of life when driver's training begins, yet parents may not trust that their ADHD adolescents are cognitively or emotionally ready to assume that level of responsibility (11). This presents families with one more issue over which to argue.

Socially, the adolescent with ADHD may continue to struggle with being accepted by peers. Conversely, they may start developing friendships, but these are commonly with adolescents who are also disinterested, unmotivated or troubled in some way. During this time there is an increased risk of becoming involved in drug and/or alcohol use. Their future goals may be vague, unrealistic (e.g., wanting to go to college as they're failing in high school), or non-existent. For families at this stage of their evolution, there are three possible responses to the situation: (1) Increasing their efforts to secure educational and therapeutic help for their ADHD adolescents; (2) Acquiescing to the adolescents, who essentially become "free boarders" in the home; or, (3) Expelling the adolescents once their legal obligations to care for them are met.

ADHD in college-age young adults (12-14)

The transition from high school to college can be challenging for students with ADHD. Studies have found that young adults with ADHD are less successful at adjusting to the demands of college than are same-age, non-ADHD peers. The adjustment difficulties are not confined to academics, as those with ADHD also struggle in the area of socialization (15). One mediating factor seems to be low self-esteem, which may have never been clinically addressed in the student's earlier years. Students with ADHD are more likely to earn lower grades, be on academic probation, and not complete college than are matched peers without ADHD. The risk of substance abuse increases even more at this time, as there is more ready access to alcohol and street drugs. An especial concern is the potential misuse or sale of the students' prescribed stimulant medications (16).

For the young adults with ADHD who forgo- or drop out of- college, life can continue to be difficult. These young people are more likely to become, or remain, unemployed. Those who do work may do so at lower wages (based mostly on lack of educational achievement), and are more likely to remain at lower job levels. Marital (and other romantic relationship) instability is not uncommon. Continued impulsivity and risk-taking behaviors can lead to motor vehicle accidents (11), gambling problems (17), and involvement with the legal system, especially if there is comorbid conduct disorder or antisocial personality disorder.

DIAGNOSIS

The following section will discuss other clinical conditions that can mimic or co-exist with ADHD. The first question to ask when presented with a child, adolescent, or young adult who is inattentive, hyperactive and/or impulsive is whether or not the symptoms are due to the direct effects of substances of abuse. Table 2 lists the classes of drugs which can be obtained both legally and illegally, and which can produce ADHD-like effects. Drugs which stimulate the CNS, such as amphetamines and cocaine, can cause motor/verbal over-activity and risk-taking that mimics hyperactivity and impulsivity, respectively. Conversely, when those drugs wear-off the person may have slowed mentation that can look like inattention. Drugs which suppress the CNS, such as anxiolytics and opiates, can make people less aware of their environments and can look like inattention; the removal of those agents can cause agitation that looks like hyperactivity.

Table 2. Substance-related* differential diagnosis for ADHD

Alcohol
Amphetamines
Anxiolytics
Caffeine
Cannabis
Cocaine
Hallucinogens
Inhalants
Opiates

* Intoxication and/or withdrawal effects.

Table 3. Medical differential diagnosis for ADHD

Neurologic disorder	Seizure disorders
	Traumatic brain injury
	Encephalitis
	Sleep disorders
Endocrine disorders	Hypothyroidism
Metabolic disorders	Diabetes mellitus
Hematologic disorders	Anemia
Cardiovascular disorders	Congenital heart disease
Gastrointestinal disorders	Celiac disease
Renal disorders	Chronic renal failure
Pulmonary disorders	Asthma
Gynecologic disorders	Premenstrual syndrome
Infectious diseases	Epstein-Barr virus infection
	Cytomegalovirus infection
	HIV infection
	Lyme disease
Toxicologic disorders	Lead poisoning
	Carbon monoxide poisoning (chronic)
Sensory disorders	Hearing impairment
	Vision impairment
Nutritional disorders	Malnutrition
Medical treatments	Brain irradiation
	Cancer chemotherapy
Medications	Antiepileptic drugs
	Corticosteroids
	Beta-adrenergic agonists
	Antibiotics
	Antidepressants
	Antipsychotics
	Lithium
	Benzodiazepines

The second question to ask is whether the ADHD-like symptoms are due to the direct effects of a medical illness or of prescription medications. Table 3 lists some of the more common medical conditions and medications that can present with features of ADHD, especially inattention and mental disorganization.

The third question to ask is whether the inattention, hyperactivity and/or impulsivity can be better accounted for by another psychiatric disorder. Table 4 lists the psychiatric diagnoses that may share features with or mimic ADHD (the reader is asked to consult the other chapters in this book for details on the diagnosis of non-ADHD psychiatric disorders).

Lastly, even when the diagnosis of ADHD can be made with certainty (see the end of this section), the clinician should look for and rule-out comorbid psychiatric disorders, the prevalence of which has been estimated at between 50% and 90% in ADHD patients (18). The importance of identifying other psychiatric issues is in their relevance to treatment and prognosis. The conditions that most commonly coexist with ADHD are:

- *Disruptive behavior disorders: Oppositional defiant disorder (ODD) and conduct disorder (CD).* In younger patients with ADHD, 30%-60% will have ODD, 20%-30% will have CD, and about 50% will have ODD and/or CD.
- *Major depressive disorder (MDD).* Having ADHD greatly increases the risk for developing depression in both males and females. Between 5% and 40% of ADHD patients will also be depressed.
- *Bipolar disorder.* There is somewhat of a bidirectional association between ADHD and bipolar disorder, in that 10%-22% of ADHD patients will eventually meet criteria for bipolar illness, while patients who are diagnosed with bipolar disorder will also have ADHD 29%-98% of the time.
- *Anxiety disorders.* In the primary pediatric setting about 50% of children with ADHD also have an anxiety disorder; conversely, 20% of children with an anxiety disorder have comorbid ADHD.
- *Tic disorders.* Large-scale epidemiological surveys have found that 50% of those with a tic disorder meet criteria for ADHD. Conversely, about 20% of those with ADHD will have some type of tic disorder.
- *Substance-use disorders (SUD).* There has been some debate regarding whether or not ADHD is an independent risk factor for the development of SUD. It seems fairly clear now that patients with ADHD are at greater risk of developing SUD if they are also comorbid for CD or bipolar disorder.
- *Learning disorders.* The academic struggles of children with ADHD could very well derive from their inattention and disorganization. However, learning disorders may coexist in as many as 70% of students with ADHD.
- *Enuresis.* Several studies have reported rates of enuresis in children with ADHD from 21% to 32%, an up to 6-fold increase compared to controls. Family studies have shown, however, that both conditions are transmitted independently of each other.
- *Sleep disorders.* Almost 50% of parents of ADHD children report that the youngsters have difficulty falling asleep and staying asleep. In addition, up to 25% will have sleep-disordered breathing and up to 36% will have excessive limb movements, including restless legs syndrome.

- *Eating disorders.* When compared to controls, girls with ADHD-C and ADHD-I have higher rates of body dissatisfaction and engage in more binge-purge behaviors. The ADHD-C girls also have higher rates of eating pathology than do the ADHD-I girls, likely related to a higher degree of impulsivity.

Table 4. Psychiatric differential diagnosis for ADHD

Developmental disorders	Intellectual disabilities
	Learning disorders
	Communication disorders
	Autism spectrum disorders
Disruptive behavior disorders	Oppositional defiant disorder
	Conduct disorder
Tic disorders	Tourette's disorder
Psychotic disorders	Schizophrenia
	Brief psychotic disorder
Mood disorders	Major depression
	Dysthymic disorder
	Bipolar disorder
	Cyclothymic disorder
Anxiety disorders	Panic disorder
	Social anxiety disorder
	Generalized anxiety disorder
Obsessive-compulsive & related disorders	Obsessive-compulsive disorder
Trauma- and stressor related disorders	Post-traumatic stress disorder
	Reactive attachment disorder
Dissociative disorders	Dissociative amnesia
Eating disorders	Anorexia nervosa
	Bulimia nervosa
Adjustment disorders	With depressed mood
	With anxiety
	With mixed anxiety and depressed mood

The diagnostic process for ADHD. This should begin with the taking of a thorough history of symptoms and behaviors, and how they are affecting development and functioning (19). The symptoms of ADHD occur in a least two settings, so feedback will need to be obtained from family members as well as those outside the home (e.g., daycare, preschool, school, youth group, etc.). The information received will be most helpful if it is in two formats: structured, formal feedback as elicited by ADHD questionnaires and rating scales (20) (a commonly used teacher rating scale is available for free at the Bright Futures website (21, 22)); and, unstructured narratives, such as notes from teachers. In patients who are of school-age their report cards should be reviewed. As previously noted regarding Tables 2-4, the interview process should inquire about substance abuse, medical illnesses, medications, and non-ADHD psychiatric symptoms. Sometimes the data is equivocal and the diagnosis unclear. In that case the patient should be referred to a clinical psychologist for more formal assessment procedures, such as computerized evaluation of attention and impulse control. Future evaluations may include functional neuroimaging (23).

Once the diagnosis of ADHD is established, an individualized treatment approach is discussed with the patient and his/her caregivers, keeping in mind potential barriers to effective treatment, such as a history of non-compliance, restrictive insurance formularies, hypersensitivity to medications, psychiatric comorbidity, and/or medical conditions or medications that may limit or interfere with the use of ADHD medications.

Table 5. Methylphenidate (MPH) preparations: Racemic mixture (*d-* & *l-* isomers)

Trade name	Forms (mg)	Dosing Schedule Start (daily)	Titration/wk	Maximum/d	Duration of effect (hrs)
Ritalin (& generics)	Tabs [S] (5, 10, 20)	5 mg, 2-3x	5-10 mg	60 mg	3-4
Methylin	Tabs [S] (5, 10, 20) Tabs [C] (2.5, 5, 10) Solution: 5 mg/ml or 10 mg/ml	5 mg, 2-3x	5-10 mg	60 mg	4-8
Ritalin SR	Tabs [SR] (20)	20 mg in the morning†	20 mg	60 mg	6-8
Metadate ER	Tabs [ER] (10, 20)	10 mg in the morning†	10 mg	60 mg	4-8
Methylin ER	Tabs [ER] (10, 20)	10 mg in the morning†	10 mg	60 mg	4-8
Metadate CD	Caps* [ER] (10, 20, 30)	20 mg in the morning†	10-20 mg	60 mg	4-8
Ritalin LA	Caps* [LA] (10, 20, 30, 40)	20 mg in the morning†	10 mg	60 mg	8-10
Concerta	Tabs [ER] (18, 27, 36, 54)	18 mg in the morning†	18 mg	54 mg in children; 72 mg in adolescents	8-12
Daytrana	Patch [TD] (10, 15, 20, 30)	10 mg, 2 hrs before effect needed; remove 9 hrs later	10 mg	30 mg	12
Quillivant	Extended-release oral suspension: 5 mg/ml	20 mg in the morning	10-20 mg	60 mg	8-12

Legend: [S] = scored; [C] = chewable; [SR]= sustained release; [ER] = extended release; [LA] = long acting; [TD] = transdermal.
* = may be sprinkled onto soft food.
† = may need to use a 2nd PM dose.

Table 6. Amphetamine preparations: Mixed salts and methamphetamine

		Dosing Schedule			Duration of effect (hrs)
Trade name	Forms (mg)	Start (daily)	Titration/wk	Maximum/d	
Adderall (& generics) [MAS]	Tabs (5, 7.5, 10, 12.5, 15, 20, 30)	5-10 mg, 1-3x	5-10 mg	40 mg	4-6
Adderall XR [MAS]	Caps* [ER] (5, 10, 15, 20, 25, 30)	5-10 mg in the morning†	5-10 mg	30 mg	8-12
Desoxyn§	Tabs (5)	5 mg, 1-3x	5 mg	25 mg	4-6

Legend: [ER]= extended release; [MAS]= mixed amphetamine salts.
* = may be sprinkled onto soft food; § = not a first-line agent (see text for comments).
† = may need to use a 2nd PM dose.

TREATMENT

The cornerstone of treatment for ADHD is the stimulant medications, which have the highest rates of efficacy of all the psychotropic medications used for ADHD. If there are no comorbid psychiatric disorders or substance use issues of concern, and after educating the patient and his/her caregiver(s) about available treatments, pharmacotherapy is initiated using either methylphenidate (MPH) or an amphetamine preparation, such as mixed amphetamine salts (MAS) or dextroamphetamine (DEX), depending on patient characteristics and clinical needs, as well as clinician and caregiver preferences. Starting doses and titration schedules for MPH, MAS, and DEX are given in tables 5, 6 and 7, respectively (the methamphetamine preparation Desoxyn® is not a first-line agent, and some physicians and/or caregivers may be hesitant to use it at all, given that its non-prescription, street equivalent is the highly abusable "meth.").

Most patients with ADHD will usually respond to stimulants. If the first agent chosen (e.g., MPH) is ineffective or intolerable, the second agent tried should be one that was not chosen initially (e.g., MAS or DEX). If for some reason neither MPH nor amphetamines are effective or well-tolerated, then the next recommended choice would be either a long-acting alpha2-agonist (clonidine or guanfacine), or atomoxetine, a non-stimulant, selective noradrenergic reuptake inhibitor. These agents are approved for use in ADHD, and, although not as effective as the stimulants, have reasonable efficacy and may work well in some patients who have failed stimulant trials. Table 8 lists the most commonly used non-stimulant agents for ADHD.

In the event of failed trials of alpha2-agonists or atomoxetine, the clinician is faced with several treatment options. The next choice could be one of the following: 1) dexmethylphenidate; 2) alpha2-agonist plus a stimulant; 3) atomoxetine plus a stimulant; 4) bupropion or venlafaxine; 5) a tricyclic antidepressant (TCA); or, a monoamine oxidase inhibitor (MAOI). Table 8 does not include the TCAs or MAOIs; it would be rare to have to use them, given the availability of newer agents that are safer and more effective. Dexmethylphenidate is the *d-* isomer of MPH (see table 9), and it can be effective in patients who have been partial responders to MPH at doses so high that it precludes further dosage increases.

Table 7. Amphetamine preparations: Racemic Isolate (d- isomer only)

Trade name	Forms (mg)	Dosing Schedule Start (daily)	Titration/wk	Maximum/d	Duration of effect (hrs)
Dexedrine (& generics)	Tabs (5)	5 mg, 1-3x	5 mg	40 mg	4-6
Dextrostat (& generics)	Tabs [S] (5,10)	2.5-5 mg, 1-3x	5 mg	40 mg	4-6
	Caps [ER] (5, 10, 20)	5 mg, 1-2x	5 mg	40 mg	4-6
Dexedrine Spansule	Spansules* (5, 10, 15)	5 mg in the morning†	5 mg	45 mg	6-10
Vyvanse	Caps** (20, 30, 40, 50, 60, 70)	20-30 mg in the morning†	10-20 mg	70 mg	12

Legend: [S]= scored; [ER]= extended release.

* = may be sprinkled onto soft food; **= may be opened and mixed with water; †= may need to use a 2nd PM dose.

Table 8. Non-stimulant agents

Trade name (generic)	Forms (mg)	Dosing Schedule Start (daily)	Titration	Maximum/d
Strattera (atomoxetine) [SNRI]	Caps (10, 18, 25, 40, 60, 80, 100)	≤ 70 kg: 0.5 mg/kg >70 kg: 40 mg	≤ 70 kg: After at least 3 days increase to target of 1.2 mg/kg/d, given once or divided >70 kg: After at least 3 days increase to target of 80 mg/d given once or divided	≤ 70 kg: 1.4 mg/kg or 100 mg, whichever is less >70 kg: 100 mg
Intuniv (extended-release guanfacine)	Tabs (1, 2, 3, 4)	1 mg, or 0.05-0.08 mg/kg, either morning or at bedtime	Increase by no more than 1mg/wk	4 mg, or 0.12 mg/kg
Kapvay (extended-release clonidine)	0.1, 0.2	0.1 mg at bedtime	0.1 mg/d at weekly intervals, divided bid, with the bigger dose at bedtime	0.4 mg
Wellbutrin* (bupropion) [DNRI]	Tabs (75, 100)	3 mg/kg or 75-150 mg, whichever is lower	After at least 3 days can increase to 100 mg, 2x/d	100 mg, 3x/d, with at least 6 hrs between doses
Wellbutrin SR*	Tabs (100, 150, 200)		After at least 3 days can increase to 150 mg, 2x/d	150 mg, 2x/d, with at least 8 hrs between doses
Wellbutrin XL*	Tabs (150, 300)		After at least 3 days can increase to 300 mg, 1x/d	300 mg, 1x/d, with at least 24 hrs between doses
Provigil* (modafinil)	Tabs (100, 200)	50 mg days 1 & 2	100 mg days 3-7 200 mg days 8-14, 300 mg days 15-21 400 mg day 22+	<30 kg: 300 mg ≥30 kg: 400 mg

Legend: SNRI = selective norepinephrine reuptake inhibitor; DNRI = dopamine and norepinephrine reuptake inhibitor.

* Not FDA-approved for the treatment of ADHD.

Table 9. Methylphenidate (MPH) preparations: Racemic Isolate (*d*-isomer only)

Trade name	Forms (mg)	Dosing Schedule Start (daily)	Titration/wk	Maximum/d	Duration of effect (hrs)
Focalin (dexMPH)	Tabs [S] (2.5,5,10)	2.5 mg, 1-3x	2.5 mg	30 mg	4-5
Focalin XR	Caps* [ER] (5,10)	5 mg in the morning†	5 mg	30 mg	8-12

Legend: [S]= scored; [ER]= extended release.
* = may be sprinkled onto soft food; † = may need to use a 2nd PM dose.

Table 10. Uncommon or serious side effects of ADHD medications

Medications	Adverse effects
Stimulants (MPH, MAS, DEX, dexMPH)	Weight loss Growth suppression Bruising Muscle damage Dyskinesia Hallucinations Mania Exacerbation of tics Increased heart rate and blood pressure Sudden cardiac death (in patients with clinically significant structural cardiac abnormalities, cardiomyopathy, or heart rhythm abnormalities)
Atomoxetine	Weight loss Suicidal ideation Mania Hepatotoxicity Seizures Increased heart rate and blood pressure (mostly diastolic)
Bupropion	Suicidal ideation Mania Seizures Increased blood pressure
Alpha agonists (clonidine, guanfacine)	Orthostatic hypotension Rebound hypertension Cardiac arrhythmias
Modafinil	Increased heart rate and blood pressure

MPH = methylphenidate; MAS= mixed amphetamine salts; DEX= dextroamphe-tamine; dexMPH = dexmethylphenidate.

The combination of either an alpha2-agonist or atomoxetine with a stimulant should be approached cautiously; given the theoretical synergistic effects they can have on the cardiovascular system. The use of an alpha agonist as monotherapy should be considered earlier in the treatment sequence if hyperactivity is severe, or if stimulants or atomoxetine worsen the ADHD symptoms, or provoke irritability or aggression. An off-label alternative to the stimulants is modafinil, a wakefulness-promoting agent used for narcolepsy; this agent came close to getting FDA approval for use in ADHD, but failed after a report of it causing the Stevens-Johnson syndrome (24). Another drawback is that modafinil is quite expensive, and insurance carriers are unlikely to pay for its use in ADHD.

Treating ADHD in the presence of comorbid conditions

At first glance this may seem like a daunting clinical task. However, the therapeutic strategy is relatively simple: first treat the disorder that is causing the most distress, is causing the most functional impairment, is the most likely to progress more quickly without treatment, and/or is associated with the worst outcome if left untreated. For example, in a child or adolescent with both ADHD and MDD, treating the depression would take priority, as the worst outcome for not treating the depressed mood (i.e., suicide) would be more serious than the worst outcomes associated with not treating the ADHD, at least in the short-term. One could consider starting with bupropion or venlafaxine, which would treat the depression and may adequately treat the ADHD symptoms. Even though atomoxetine is a selective noradrenergic reuptake inhibitor, and theoretically should act as an antidepressant, in reality it shows poor antidepressant effects in pediatric patients. The TCAs, likewise, are not effective antidepressants in depressed youth. Some experts recommend treating the ADHD first, as some comorbid symptoms (e.g., depression, anxiety, or even irritability (25)) may improve coincidentally with the improvement in ADHD. An argument can be made against that strategy, as it's also possible that comorbid problems (including depression, anxiety, anger, mania and/or tics) could be exacerbated by the medications used to treat ADHD. If stimulant medications are used as first-line agents to treat ADHD comorbid with another psychiatric disorder, patients should be monitored closely for exacerbation of either condition.

Medication side effects

The adverse effects associated with medications for ADHD are usually transient and not severe (26). The most common side effects from the stimulants are headaches, stomachaches, decreased appetite, insomnia and irritability. Atomoxetine tends to produce more gastrointestinal (GI) symptoms than do the stimulants and may also cause fatigue. Bupropion causes side effects similar to the stimulants, but generally to a greater degree. The alpha agonists mostly cause sedation, and may need to be taken at nighttime; hypotension is less common in pediatric patients. The side effects from modafinil commonly derive from the GI and nervous systems. More serious adverse effects are listed in table 10 (see (27) for a more detailed discussion).

As can be seen in table 10, although not common, the medications used for ADHD can have effects on the cardiovascular system (28); this is especially of concern in those with preexisting cardiac abnormalities or other cardiac risk factors, such as a positive family history of early cardiac disease or death. All children who are to be started on ADHD medications should have baseline pulse and blood pressure recorded, and those parameters should be monitored at each visit. Routine ECGs are not recommended, but can be obtained on selected patients when clinically appropriate (29).

Complementary and alternative medical therapies for ADHD

For some parents, the possibility of their children experiencing any of the aforementioned side effects is unacceptable. This is a fairly common reason that some parents seek out more "natural" treatments for ADHD, such as complementary and alternative medical therapies (CAM). An analysis of data from a 2007 national survey of youth (7-17 years old) found that in those with ADHD, 24.7% had tried at least one form of CAM (30). The most frequently used modalities were: mind-body practices (e.g., biofeedback, hypnosis), 15.0%; biologically based therapies (e.g., diet, dietary supplements), 9.3%; and, manipulation and body-based practices (e.g., chiropractic/osteopathic, massage), 6.6%.

In recent years there has been an increase in research on the use of CAM for psychiatric disorders, including ADHD. Unfortunately, many of the studies are not of good quality, leaving clinicians and the public with little to help them make informed decisions about the use of CAM for their respective patients and children. Despite those limitations, there are some indications that, in some patients, the motor and/or cognitive symptoms of ADHD can be improved by physical activity (31), an elimination diet (32), neurofeedback (33), polyunsaturated fatty acids (34, 35) and *Ginkgo biloba* (36).

CONCLUSION

This review has discussed attention-deficit/hyperactivity disorder (ADHD) in terms of definition, epidemiology, diagnosis, comorbidity and treatment. It is hoped that the information contained herein will be helpful to pediatricians in the management of their patients with ADHD. More detailed information can be found in the bibliographic references.

REFERENCES

[1] Efron D. Attention-deficit/hyperactivity disorder: the past 50 years. J Paediatr Child Health 2015;51(1):69-73.
[2] Kieling C, Kieling R, Rohde LA, Frick PJ, Moffitt T, Nigg J, Tannock R, Castellanos FX. The age-at-onset of ADHD. Am J Psychiatry 2010;167(1):14-6.
[3] American Psychiatric Association. Diagnostic and statistical manual of mental disorders (DSM-5). Arlington, VA: American Psychiatric Association, 2013.
[4] Skounti M, Philalithis A, Galanakis E. Variations in prevalence of attention deficit hyperactivity disorder worldwide. Eur J Pediatr 2007;166(2):117-23.
[5] Polanczyk G, de Lima MS, Horta BL, Biederman J, Rohde LA. The worldwide prevalence of ADHD: a systematic review and metaregression analysis. Am J Psychiatry 2007;164(6):942-8.

[6] Hervey-Jumper H, Douyon K, Falcone T, Franco KN. Identifying, evaluating, diagnosing, and treating ADHD in minority youth. J Atten Disord 2008;11(5):522-8.
[7] Naglieri JA, Goldstein S. The role of intellectual processes in the DSM-V diagnosis of ADHD. J Atten Disord 2006;10(1):3-8.
[8] Posner K, Melvin GA, Murray DW, Gugga SS, Fisher P, Skrobala A, et al. Clinical presentation of attention-deficit/hyperactivity disorder in preschool children: the Preschoolers with Attention-Deficit/Hyperactivity Disorder Treatment Study (PATS). J Child Adolesc Psychopharmacol 2007;17(5):547-62.
[9] Morrow RL, Garland EJ, Wright JM, Maclure M, Taylor S, Dormuth CR. Influence of relative age on diagnosis and treatment of attention-deficit/hyperactivity disorder in children. CMAJ 2012;184(7):755-62.
[10] Hurtig T, Ebeling H, Taanila A, Miettunen J, Smalley SL, McGough JJ, et al. ADHD symptoms and subtypes: relationship between childhood and adolescent symptoms. J Am Acad Child Adolesc Psychiatry 2007;46(12):1605-13.
[11] Thompson AL, Molina BS, Pelham W Jr, Gnagy EM. Risky driving in adolescents and young adults with childhood ADHD. J Pediatr Psychol 2007;32(7):745-59.
[12] Sacchetti GM, Lefler EK. ADHD symptomology and social functioning in college students. J Atten Disord 2014 Nov 17. pii: 1087054714557355.
[13] Shaw-Zirt B, Popali-Lehane L, Chaplin W, Bergman A. Adjustment, social skills, and self-esteem in college students with symptoms of ADHD. J Atten Disord 2005;8(3):109-20.
[14] Wolf LE, Simkowitz P, Carlson H. College students with attention-deficit/hyperactivity disorder. Curr Psychiatry Rep 2009;11(5):415-21.
[15] Green AL, Rabiner DL. What do we really know about ADHD in college students? Neurotherapeutics 2012;98(3):559-68.
[16] Benson K, Flory K, Humphreys KL, Lee SS. Misuse of stimulant medication among college students: a comprehensive review and meta-analysis. Clin Child Fam Psychol Rev 2015;18(1):50-76.
[17] Grall-Bronnec M, Wainstein L, Augy J, Bouju G, Feuillet F, Vénisse JL, Sébille-Rivain V. Attention deficit hyperactivity disorder among pathological and at-risk gamblers seeking treatment: a hidden disorder. Eur Addict Res 2011;17(5):231-40.
[18] Kunwar A, Dewan M, Faraone SV. Treating common psychiatric disorders associated with attention-deficit/hyperactivity disorder. Expert Opin Pharmacother 2007;8(5):555-62.
[19] Pliszka S; AACAP Work Group on Quality Issues. Practice parameter for the assessment and treatment of children and adolescents with Attention-Deficit/Hyperactivity Disorder. J Am Acad Child Adolesc Psychiatry 2007; 46(7):894-921.
[20] Pelham WE Jr, Fabiano GA, Massetti GM. Evidence-based assessment of attention deficit hyperactivity disorder in children and adolescents. J Clin Child Adolesc Psychol 2005;34(3):449-76.
[21] Bright Futures in Practice: Mental Health-Volume I, Practice Guide. Attention Deficit Hyperactivity Disorder. URL: http://www.brightfutures.org/ mentalhealth/pdf/bridges/ adhd.pdf
[22] Bright Futures in Practice: Mental Health-Volume II, Tool Kit. Vanderbilt ADHD Diagnostic Teacher Rating Scale. URL: http://www.brightfutures.org/mentalhealth/ pdf/professionals/bridges/adhd.pdf
[23] Iannaccone R, Hauser TU, Ball J, Brandeis D, Walitza S, Brem S. Classifying adolescent attention-deficit/hyperactivity disorder (ADHD) based on functional and structural imaging. Eur Child Adolesc Psychiatr 2015 Jan 23.
[24] Manos MJ, Tom-Revzon C, Bukstein OG, Crismon ML. Changes and challenges: managing ADHD in a fast-paced world. J Manag Care Pharm 2007;13(9 Suppl B):S2-S13.
[25] Fernández de la Cruz L, Simonoff E, McGough JJ, Halperin JM, Arnold LE, Stringaris A. Treatment of children with attention-deficit/hyperactivity disorder (ADHD) and irritability: Results from the Multimodal Treatment Sutud of Children with ADHD (MTA). J Am Acad Child Adolesc Psychiatr 2015;54(1):62-70.
[26] Himpel S, Banaschewski T, Heise CA, Rothenberger A. The safety of non-stimulant agents for the treatment of attention-deficit hyperactivity disorder. Expert Opin Drug Saf 2005;4(2):311-21.
[27] Wolraich ML, McGuinn L, Doffing M. Treatment of attention deficit hyperactivity disorder in children and adolescents: safety considerations. Drug Saf 2007;30(1):17-26.

[28] Vitiello B. Understanding the risk of using medications for attention deficit hyperactivity disorder with respect to physical growth and cardiovascular function. Child Adolesc Psychiatric Clin N Am 2008;17:459-74.
[29] Daughton J, Liu H, West M, Swanson D, Kratochvil CJ. Practical guide to ADHD pharmacotherapy. Psychiatr Ann 2010;40(4):210-7.
[30] Kemper KJ, Gardiner P, Birdee GS. Use of complementary and alternative medical therapies among youth with mental health concerns. Acad Pediatr 2013;13(6):540-5.
[31] Ziereis S, Jansen P. Effects of physical activity on executive function and motor performance in children with ADHD. Res Dev Disabil 2015;38:181-91.
[32] Nigg JT, Holton K. Restriction and elimination diets in ADHD treatment. Child Adolesc Psychiatr Clin North Am 2014;23(4):937-53.
[33] Duric NS, Aßmus J, Elgen IB. Self-reported efficacy of neurofeedback treatment in a clinical randomized controlled study of ADHD children and adolescents. Neuropsychiatr Dis Treat 2014;10:1645-54.
[34] Bloch MH, Mulqueen J. Nutritional supplements for the treatment of ADHD. Child Adolesc Psychiatr Clin North Am 2014;23(4):883-97.
[35] Puri BK, Martins JG. Which polyunsaturated fatty acids are active in children with attention-deficit hyperactivity disorder receiving PUFA supplementation? A fatty acid validated meta-regression analysis of randomized controlled trials. Prostaglandins Leukot Essent Fatty Acids 2014;90(5):179-89.
[36] Shakibaei F, Radmanesh M, Salari E, Mahaki B. Ginkgo biloba in the treatment of attention-deficit/hyperactivity disorder in children and adolescents. A randomized, placebo-controlled trial. Complement Ther Clin Pract 2015;21(2):61-7.

In: Mental and Holistic Health: Some International Perspectives   ISBN: 978-1-63483-589-3
Editors: J. Calles Jr., D. Greydanus and J. Merrick   © 2015 Nova Science Publishers, Inc.

Chapter 3

NEUROPSYCHIATRIC DISORDERS: OPPOSITIONAL DEFIANT AND CONDUCT DISORDERS

Joseph L Calles Jr.[*], *MD*

Department of Psychiatry, Western Michigan University Homer Stryker MD School of Medicine, Kalamazoo, Michigan, United States

Oppositional defiant disorder (ODD) and conduct disorder (CD) are commonly encountered in psychiatric and legal settings, yet they can be missed, or attributed to other conditions, in general pediatric settings. This review will describe the clinical features of oppositional defiant disorder and conduct disorder, and discuss treatment options, including selected complementary and alternative interventions. The successful diagnosis and treatment of patients with ODD and CD is dependent on identifying and treating comorbid psychiatric disorders, initiating multidisciplinary psychosocial interventions, and reasoned engagement of the legal system. The primary pediatrician is in the position to serve as the gateway through which patients and their families can be directed to the necessary community resources. The pediatrician may also choose to prescribe and manage the patients' medications.

INTRODUCTION

It is fairly common for clinicians to have contact with younger patients who are resistant, provocative, challenging, non-communicative and/or hostile. They may also be non-compliant with medical recommendations. In the office setting, they can divert an inordinate amount of time and energy away from other patients. They are described by their tired and frustrated parents as being the same way at home and sometimes at school. These children and adolescents who are diagnosed with oppositional defiant disorder or conduct disorder can elicit feelings of anger on the part of the physician, potentially compromising the quality of medical care. In order to provide effective treatment, it is important that the physician not only document the behaviors, but look beyond them and assess for psychopathology that is

---

[*] Correspondence: Professor Joseph L Calles Jr, Department of Psychiatry, Western Michigan University Homer Stryker M.D. School of Medicine, 1717 Shaffer Road, Suite 010, Kalamazoo, MI 49048, United States. E-mail: joseph.calles@med.wmich.edu.

likely to be driving the behaviors. What follows is a discussion of the epidemiology, core clinical features, and treatment recommendations of both disorders.

DEFINITION

In the most recent (fifth) edition of the American Psychiatric Association's "Diagnostic and statistical manual of mental disorders (DSM-5)" (1), one section is entitled "disruptive, impulse-control, and conduct disorders." The two most common disorders described in that section are oppositional defiant disorder and conduct disorder (2) (disruptive behavior disorders (DBDs), in general, will be discussed in the chapter on Aggressive Behaviors).

Oppositional defiant disorder (ODD) is characterized by a pattern of angry or irritable mood, argumentative or defiant behavior, or vindictiveness in children or adolescents, often in response to rules, requests, or expectations initiated by others (excluding siblings), usually authority figures, of at least 6-months duration. The anger can be expressed directly through arguments or willful annoyance of others; its indirect expression can take the form of vindictiveness ("payback"). The behavior is usually confined to the home, and may never be displayed in other settings, although it is not uncommon to see ODD children "tantrum" in public settings when they don't get what they want. It should be kept in mind that all children exhibit these types of behaviors at some point, and that it is the persistence, frequency and severity of the behaviors that distinguish the "normal" from the pathologic. These behaviors do not occur exclusively during the course of another psychiatric disorder.

Conduct disorder (CD) describes a set of behaviors (at least 3 within the past 12 months, and at least 1 present in the last 6 months) that are more serious, in intentions and consequences, than those seen in ODD. In addition to rules, children and adolescents with CD display aggression towards other living beings (people, pets), are destructive of property, lie and steal, and seriously violate rules (e.g., staying out past curfew, running away, and/or being truant from school). Covert symptoms (e.g., stealing) may never be discovered; overt symptoms (e.g., fighting) are difficult to ignore. The childhood-onset type is distinguished from the adolescent-onset type by whether at least one characteristic symptom was present before or after the age of 10 years, respectively. A more serious subtype of CD (seen in about 21% to 50% of clinic-referred CD) is seen in those with *callous-unemotional* (CU) traits (3). Those individuals are characterized as having low levels of fear, as well as a lack of empathy, guilt, and emotion. What is significant about this subtype is that it is associated with poorer outcomes, which includes higher rates of substance abuse, violent offending, criminal activity and psychopathy, s higher genetic risk factors.

EPIDEMIOLOGY

Prevalence studies of ODD and CD can produce data that are quite variable and contradictory. Results can be influenced by the populations sampled, the ages and developmental levels of the subjects, and diagnostic criteria and/or instruments used. A review of international studies of the estimated prevalence of ODD and CD did not find any significant variability in rates based on geographic location (which may be a proxy for

Oppositional defiant disorder

Although the data are scant regarding ODD in very young children, one study (5) found that in children ages 3 to 5 years referred to a psychiatric specialty clinic for preschool behavior problems, ODD symptoms were seen in 31.6% to 72.2% (as compared to 0.0% to 8.0% in the non-referred comparison group). The actual rates of ODD diagnosis in the two groups were 59.5% vs. 2.0%, respectively.

It is unclear whether increasing age affects the prevalence of ODD in the general population, although there does seem to be a decrease over time (6). However, the rate of ODD symptoms stays fairly steady as children get older *if* there is significant overlap with CD symptoms.

Conduct disorder

The preschool study (5) that looked at ODD symptoms also investigated the presence of CD symptoms, which were highly variable but significant in the referred population, ranging from 2.5% to 44.9% (but ≤ 4.0% in the non-referred sample). The rate of CD diagnosis in the two groups was likewise discrepant, made in 41.8% vs. 2.0%, respectively.

The relationship between aging and CD is more certain than that of ODD and aging, at least as far as the CD behaviors that are also seen in juvenile delinquents. There seems to be an increase of covert (non-aggressive) conduct behaviors, a decrease in minor aggression (e.g., fighting), and an increase in major aggression (e.g., rape and murder) into and through adolescence (6).

CLINICAL FEATURES

Oppositional defiant disorder

As previously mentioned, children and adolescents with ODD have major issues with rules and authority figures. In some sense ODD behaviors are an exaggeration and a prolongation of the normal developmental resistance seen in toddlers ("the terrible twos"), and parents often tell us that their ODD child has been "stubborn from the beginning." The tantrums that begin in early life are disruptive to the family, and also cause concern of inadvertent injury to the child. As the child gets older, bigger, and stronger, the concern of injury to family members develops. Even though the child or adolescent may not have been, or may never be, physically aggressive towards others in the home, it is the *possibility* of violence that often keeps parents from disciplining in ways that they would ordinarily use, thus reinforcing the behavior. This is especially true when the angry individual aggressively acts out against property, e.g., punching holes in the wall, throwing and breaking things, etc., and are not made to clean up, repair, and/or replace the damaged objects.

It is almost guaranteed that the ODD child or adolescent will become angry when their wishes, desires, or expectations are frustrated (in other words, when they are told "no"). He/she will often react by yelling, swearing, or threatening to harm others (or occasionally himself/herself). The adults may be accused of "not caring" or "not understanding" their child and they may be unfavorably compared to friends' parents, who reportedly let their children "do what they want." The other common cause of conflicts is when the children or adolescents do not follow through on what is expected of them (e.g., chores; homework). This is often compounded by their lying to avoid the task itself ("I didn't have any homework"), or to avoid the consequences for not doing the task ("I didn't cut the grass because the mower is broken"). Lying can also be combined with blame, such that the work that is not done is made to seem the fault of the parent, not the child ("You didn't tell me that you wanted it done today!").

Youth with ODD resent being called on their behaviors and having negative consequences. They may engage in spiteful behaviors that range from the relatively trivial (e.g., coming home late, thus missing their doctor's appointment) to the potentially more serious (e.g., making false accusations of parental abuse).

Conduct disorder

In preschool children, disruptive behavioral markers can be identified not only for current CD, but for later school-age CD (7). Boys with CD like to fight and can do so with minimal-to-no provocation. Some of them have a high tolerance for pain, so their own discomfort may not stop them from hurting someone to the point of serious injury (e.g., fractured jaw), unconsciousness, or even death. They also don't like to lose, so they may employ weapons during a fight, thus increasing the potential of damage to others. The threat of violence can also be used to steal money (e.g., armed robbery) or to sexually violate someone, i.e., rape. The hurting of others for pleasure can extend to animals, with the possible end-result being the death of the animal. One of the more bothersome aspects of CD is that some youth with it seem to have no remorse for their harmful acts, and may even rationalize them ("He deserved it because he was disrespecting me"). The lack of remorse, lack of empathy, lack of concern about performance (school, work, other important activities), and/or shallow or insincere affect have been termed *callous-unemotional traits*, and, when present, are associated with higher levels of aggression and cruelty (8).

Some boys also engage in destructive behaviors "for the fun of it," or because they're "bored." Arson is the most serious and dangerous manifestation of this, but malicious destruction of property- breaking windows, painting graffiti, tearing up landscaping- can lead to large repair bills for homeowners, businesses and government agencies.

Boys and girls with CD may both lie and steal to get what they want. Boys tend to use more extreme methods, such as breaking and entering ("B&E") into buildings or stealing a car (grand theft auto ("GTA")). Girls tend to employ more subtle techniques, such as shoplifting, running up large bills on a parent's credit card, or manipulating male friends to steal for them.

Running away and skipping school are ways for the CD child or adolescent to avoid responsibilities and to seek out excitement. They also place the person at risk of getting involved in dangerous activities, such as unprotected sex or substance use, criminal behaviors, or becoming victims of violence themselves.

Parents may be hesitant to engage law enforcement agencies or to file legal charges, in the belief that doing so will "ruin" their child's future (9). They tend to not realize that, in the absence of meaningful negative consequences, their child is more likely to continue in their maladaptive behaviors, increasing the likelihood of eventual contact with the criminal justice system. Parents need to understand that the time to intervene is early, when they have a say in what happens to their child. If parents act too late, the legal system will be the sole arbiter of outcome.

DIAGNOSIS

Oppositional defiant disorder

The identification of ODD is usually straight-forward, based on observable behavioral criteria; however, two cautions are necessary in that regard. The first is that oppositional behaviors may derive from other psychiatric disorders, may be a transient response to stressors, or may be part of normal developmental stages (Table 1). The second is that ODD usually does not exist in isolation from other psychiatric disorders, so it is important to search for and identify other potentially treatable comorbid conditions (10).

Table 1. Other conditions that may present with oppositional/defiant behaviors

Normal toddlerhood or early adolescence
Intellectual disabilities
Neurodevelopmental disorders
• Attention-deficit/hyperactivity disorder
• Autism spectrum disorder
• Communication disorders
Disruptive disorders (other than ODD)
• Conduct disorder
• Intermittent explosive disorder
Mood disorders
• Major depressive disorder
• Persistent depressive (dysthymic) disorder
• Bipolar disorder
• Disruptive mood dysregulation disorder
Psychotic disorders
Substance-use disorders
Adjustment disorders
Medical disorders, especially neurologic disorders

The most common disorder comorbid with ODD is attention-deficit/hyperactivity disorder (ADHD). The presence of hyperactive-impulsive symptoms actually predisposes to the development of ODD (11); in one study of 3-7 year-olds with combined type ADHD, a full 60% also met criteria for ODD (12). Therefore, when either ADHD or ODD is diagnosed, the clinician should always rule-out the presence of the other (see the chapter on Attention-deficit/hyperactivity disorder for details).

Clinically-referred patients with ODD also have significant rates of comorbid major depressive disorder (MDD), bipolar disorder (BD), and multiple anxiety disorders (MA) when compared to patients with psychiatric disorders other than ODD (or CD). When the group with other diagnoses was assessed, high rates of ODD were found in those with ADHD, MDD, BD, pervasive developmental disorders, MA, Tourette's disorder, and language disorders. Adolescents with ODD are also at risk for developing alcohol dependence by adulthood (13).

Conduct disorder

The same cautions noted for ODD, regarding conditions that may mimic or be comorbid with the disorder (e.g., ADHD (14)), also apply to CD (see table 1). In children or adolescents who display isolated (not pervasive) conduct problems that do not meet criteria for CD or adjustment disorder with disturbance of conduct, the diagnosis of an unspecified disruptive disorder may be made.

Conduct disorder is highly comorbid with any disorder of mood, anxiety (except agoraphobia), impulse control, or substance use (15) when compared to the general population. Conduct disorder is likely to develop before mood disorders about 70% of the time and before substance use disorders almost 89% of the time (16). Conversely, CD is more likely to develop after other disorders with impulsivity (e.g., ADHD and/or ODD) about 23% of the time. The temporal relationship between CD and anxiety disorders is mixed, with CD occurring after specific and social phobias but before all the other anxiety disorders about 32% of the time.

Diagnostic dilemmas

In the older Diagnostic and Statistical Manual of Mental Disorders, Fourth Edition, Text Revision (17), the diagnosis of ODD could not be made if criteria were met for CD; however, in the real world the two conditions often coexist. For example, in a longitudinal community study (18) the majority of boys with CD also showed oppositional features, and one-quarter met full criteria for ODD. Interestingly, among the girls that were assessed, there was a stronger degree of overlap, with slightly over one-half of the girls with CD also meeting full ODD criteria. There was a reverse correlation between ODD and CD symptoms, in that 57% of boys and 55% of girls with ODD also evidenced substantial (but sub-diagnostic) levels of CD symptomatology. Based on the research that confirms the high degree of overlap between ODD and CD, the cross-diagnostic exclusion has been eliminated from the new DSM-5.

Psychodiagnostic assessment

Given the high degrees of comorbidity in both ODD and CD, and the high degree of overlap between ODD and CD symptoms, accurately identifying all of the psychiatric disorders in any given patient can be challenging. The task can be nearly impossible if the patient and parent/guardian are unreliable historians. The use of standardized questionnaires and rating scales, structured or semi-structured interviews, validated observation protocols, and/or age-appropriate psychological testing can often be helpful in answering difficult clinical questions. As many of these methods require both time and specialized training, the pediatrician should enlist the consultative skills of, or refer to, a clinical psychologist as early in the process as possible (see the chapter 3 on behavioral and psychological Assessment).

TREATMENT

Oppositional defiant disorder

Good outcomes in the treatment of ODD are predicated on comprehensive evaluation and individualized interventions. The American Academy of Child and Adolescent Psychiatry has issued a practice parameter in this regard (19), which is summarized in table 2. The treatment plan will likely include psychological care of the child and family, pharmacologic treatment of the child, school-based interventions, and, in more serious cases, out-of-home placement.

An essential component of the treatment plan is some form of parent management training (PMT) (20), which is based on the sound behavioral principles of: 1) reducing positive reinforcement of the undesirable behaviors (also called extinction, or the "starving" of the negative behaviors, e.g., ignoring a tantrum); 2) increasing reinforcement of desirable behaviors (i.e., paying attention to positive behaviors, or "catching them when they're good"); 3) using age-appropriate consequences that fit the behaviors (e.g., a "reward" for a younger child could be more time spent with the parent, whereas for the older child it could be having more time to pursue his/her interests. For "punishments" the younger child could be timed-out, whereas for the older child it could be the loss of privileges) and 4) responding in a consistent and non-arbitrary manner, as soon as possible after the observed behaviors.

To date there have not been any medications that have been found to be consistently effective in treating the core symptoms of ODD (21). However, it is becoming increasingly more common for clinicians to treat DBDs with atypical antipsychotics (AAs), despite the relative paucity of research in that area. There is limited evidence, in the short term (i.e., up to 6 months), that risperidone can reduce aggressive behaviors in children and adolescents (ages 5-18 years) with DBDs, especially if they are in the autism spectrum and/or have intellectual impairments (22). The major limitation in the use of risperidone is weight gain.

Clinically, there are two circumstances in which the use of medications in ODD patients would be appropriate. The first is if there are clearly identified comorbid conditions that are amenable to pharmacotherapy, such as ADHD and MDD. For example, a comparison study of atomoxetine (ATX) and guanfacine extended release (GXR) found that the latter agent was associated with a significantly greater reduction in oppositional scores in patients with comorbid ADHD and ODD (23). The second indication for the use of medications to treat

ODD is when the disruptive behaviors are unchanged, or worsening, despite good behavioral efforts. The clinician needs to remember that medications should never be the only treatment used in patients with ODD.

Table 2. Recommendations for the evaluation and treatment of ODD

1. Establishment of therapeutic alliances with the child and family.
2. Cultural issues need to be considered in diagnosis and treatment.
3. Assessment includes information obtained directly from the child and from the parents regarding the core symptoms, age of onset, duration of symptoms, and degree of functional impairment.
4. Consider significant comorbid psychiatric conditions when diagnosing and treating ODD.
5. Include, if needed, information obtained independently from multiple outside informants.
6. Specific questionnaires and rating scales may be useful in evaluating for ODD and for tracking progress.
7. Develop an individualized treatment plan based on the specific clinical issues.
8. Choose a parent intervention based on empirically tested behavioral programs.
9. Medications should be used as adjuncts, for symptomatic treatment, and to treat comorbid conditions.
10. Intensive and prolonged treatment may be necessary if ODD is unusually severe and persistent.
11. Certain interventions (such as "boot camps") are not effective, and should be avoided, as they may worsen some behaviors.

Conduct disorder

The approach to the treatment of CD is similar to that of ODD, beginning with good history-taking and mental status examination. Particular attention is paid to signs and symptoms that could indicate comorbid conditions, which can affect the response to treatments (24, 25).

For mild-moderate CD problems, it is reasonable to start with PMT (20) (as was previously discussed for ODD); although it is unclear if the positive outcomes demonstrated in research settings can be effectively translated to the "real world" of clinical practice. For more severe conduct symptoms, such as violent behavior, parents are encouraged to utilize law enforcement interventions, including the filing of formal charges against their child or adolescent when appropriate to do so. If the child or adolescent is incarcerated, the parents are advised to not bail-out their son or daughter, as the loss of freedom is a natural consequence of his/her inappropriate and illegal actions. Depending on how unsafe the parents and/or siblings feel about the offending youth returning home, alternative living situations may have to be arranged before he/she is released.

If comorbid conditions are diagnosed they are treated following the protocols discussed elsewhere in this book (e.g., the chapters on ADHD and Depressive disorders). In the absence of clearly identified comorbid psychiatric disorders and/or response to behavioral psychotherapy, medication may still be an option, although well-designed studies are limited (26).

Lithium and risperidone have been shown to reduce CD symptoms across several measures of behavior and mood; their use requires ongoing monitoring for potentially serious side effects. The psychostimulants, ATX, valproic acid, aripiprazole, the alpha-2 agonists, and the selective serotonin reuptake inhibitors (SSRIs) have also shown promise in treating CD symptoms, but larger, well-controlled research studies demonstrating efficacy and safety are needed before routine use of these agents can be recommended. Open-label studies of olanzapine (27) and clozapine (28) in youth with severe, refractory CD demonstrated significant reductions in aggressive behaviors; further investigations of these agents are needed, as well. Given the serious- and potentially life-threatening- side effects associated with the use of clozapine, it should be managed by psychiatrists who have experience using it in younger patients.

Complementary and alternative medical treatments (CAM)

This term is sometimes used to refer to non-pharmacologic interventions. As such, the mainstream psychotherapies- including the aforementioned PMT- could be included in CAM. However, most clinicians think of CAM as those therapeutic interventions that are out of the mainstream. Considering all of the approaches to treatment of ODD and CD that have been tried, two that seem to be safe and show promise are nutritional modification and structured physical activity.

A study conducted on the island nation of Mauritius found that children who were malnourished at the age of 3 years were more likely to show signs of over activity, aggression and conduct disorder by age 17 years (29). A later, unrelated study from the UK compared the effects on behavior, in young adult prisoners, of a dietary supplement (containing daily requirements of vitamins, minerals and essential fatty acids) versus placebo (30). In those who received the actual supplement, there was a significant reduction in all offenses, including serious ones such as violent behaviors. Given that the typical diets of many first-world children emphasize carbohydrates, and ignore fruits and vegetables, the use of nutritional supplements and, preferably, a healthy, balanced diet in youth with ODD or CD seems reasonable.

Regarding the use of structured physical activity, there is some evidence that martial arts training can reduce behavioral problems in young people (31). Although activities that involve actions such as punching and kicking would seem to be counterintuitive, the martial arts may derive their beneficial effects on aggression through their emphasis on mutual respect and self-discipline.

CONCLUSION

The successful diagnosis and treatment of patients with ODD and CD is dependent on identifying and treating comorbid psychiatric disorders, initiating multidisciplinary psychosocial interventions, and reasoned engagement of the legal system. The primary pediatrician is in the position to serve as the gateway through which patients and their families can be directed to the necessary community resources. The pediatrician may also choose to prescribe and manage the patients' medications.

REFERENCES

[1] American Psychiatric Association. Diagnostic and statistical manual of mental disorders, 5th ed. Washington, DC: American Psychiatric Association, 2013.
[2] Loeber R, Burke JD, Lahey BB, Winters A, Zera M. Oppositional defiant and conduct disorder: a review of the past 10 years, Part I. J Am Acad Child Adolesc Psychiatry 2000;39(12):1468-84.
[3] Kahn RE, Frick PJ, Youngstrom E, Findling RL, Youngstrom JK. The effects of including a callous-unemotional specifier for the diagnosis of conduct disorder. J Child Psychol Psychiatry 2012;53(3):271-82.
[4] Canino G, Polanczyk G, Bauermeister JJ, Rohde LA, Frick PJ. Does the prevalence of CD and ODD vary across cultures? Soc Psychiatry Psychiatr Epidemiol 2010;45(7):695-704.
[5] Keenan K, Wakschlag LS, Danis B, Hill C, Humphries M, Duax J, et al. Further evidence of the reliability and validity of DSM-IV ODD and CD in preschool children. J Am Acad Child Adolesc Psychiatry 2007;46(4):457-68.
[6] Maughan B, Rowe R, Messer J, Goodman R, Meltzer H. Conduct disorder and oppositional defiant disorder in a national sample: developmental epidemiology. J Child Psychol Psychiatry 2004;45(3):609-21.
[7] Hong JS, Tillman R, Luby JL. Disruptive behavior in preschool children: distinguishing normal misbehavior from markers of current and later childhood conduct disorder. J Pediatric 2015;166(3):723-30.
[8] Blair RJ, Leibenluft E, Pine DS. Conduct disorder and callous-unemotional traits. N Engl J Med 2014;371(23):2207-16.
[9] Freeze MK, Burke A, Vorster AC. The role of parental style in the conduct disorders: a comparison between adolescent boys with and without conduct disorder. J Child Adolesc Ment Health 2014;26(1):63-73.
[10] Greene RW, Biederman J, Zerwas S, Monuteaux MC, Goring JC, Faraone SV. Psychiatric comorbidity, family dysfunction, and social impairment in referred youth with oppositional defiant disorder. Am J Psychiatry 2002;159(7):1214-24.
[11] Burns GL, Walsh JA. The influence of ADHD-hyperactivity/impulsivity symptoms on the development of oppositional defiant disorder symptoms in a 2-year longitudinal study. J Abnorm Child Psychol 2002;30(3):245-56.
[12] Kadesjo C, Hagglof B, Kadesjo B, Gillberg C. Attention-deficit-hyperactivity disorder with and without oppositional defiant disorder in 3- to 7-year-old children. Dev Med Child Neurol 2003;45(10):693-99.
[13] Ghosh A, Malhotra S, Basu D. Oppositional defiant disorder (ODD), the forerunner of alcohol dependence: a controlled study. Asian J Psychiatr 2014;11:8-12.
[14] Rubia K. "Cool" inferior frontostriatal dysfunction in attention-deficit/hyperactivity disorder versus "hot" ventromedial orbitofrontal-limbic dysfunction in conduct disorder: a review. Biol Psychiatry 2011;69(12):e69-e87.
[15] Brinkman WB, Epstein JN, Auinger P, Tamm L, Froehlich TE. Association of attention-deficit/hyperactivity disorder and conduct disorder with early tobacco and alcohol use. Drug Alcohol Depend 2015;147:183-9.
[16] Nock MK, Kazdin AE, Hiripi E, Kessler RC. Prevalence, subtypes, and correlates of DSM- IV conduct disorder in the National Comorbidity Survey Replication. Psychol Med 2006;36(5):699-710.
[17] American Psychiatric Association. Diagnostic and statistical manual of mental disorders, 4th ed, text revision. Washington, DC: American Psychiatric Association, 2000.

[18] Rowe R, Maughan B, Pickles A, Costello EJ, Angold A. The relationship between DSM-IV oppositional defiant disorder and conduct disorder: findings from the Great Smoky Mountains Study. J Child Psychol Psychiatr 2002;43(3):365-73.

[19] Steiner H, Remsing L; Work Group on Quality Issues. Practice parameter for the assessment and treatment of children and adolescents with oppositional defiant disorder. J Am Acad Child Adolesc Psychiatry 2007;46(1):126-41.

[20] van de Wiel N, Matthys W, Cohen-Kettenis PC, van Engeland H. Effective treatments of school-aged conduct disordered children: recommendations for changing clinical and research practices. Eur Child Adolesc Psychiatry 2002;11:79-84.

[21] Ipser J, Stein DJ. Systematic review of pharmacotherapy of disruptive behavior disorders in children and adolescents. Psychopharmacol 2007;191:127-40.

[22] Loy JH, Merry SN, Hetrick SE, Stasiak K. Atypical antipsychotics for disruptive behaviour disorders in children and youths. Cochrane Database Syst Rev 2012;9:CD008559. doi:10. 1002/ 14651858.CD008559.pub2.

[23] Signorovitch J, Erder MH, Xie J, Sikirica V, Lu M, Hodgkins PS, et al. Comparative effectiveness research using matching-adjusted indirect comparison: an application to treatment with guanfacine extended release or atomoxetine in children with attention- deficit/hyperactivity disorder and comorbid oppositional defiant disorder. Pharmacoepidemiol Drug Saf 2012;21(Suppl 2):130-7.

[24] Masi G, Muratori P, Manfredi A, Lenzi F, Polidori L, Ruglioni L et al. Response to treatments in youth with disruptive behavior disorders. Compr Psychiatry 2013;54(7):1009-15.

[25] Masi G, Milone A, Paciello M, Lenzi F, Muratori P, Manfredi A et al. Efficacy of multimodal treatment for disruptive behavioral disorders in children and adolescents: focus on internalizing problems. Psychiatry Res 2014;219(3):617-24.

[26] Sarteschi CM. Randomized controlled trials of psychopharmacological interventions of children and adolescents with conduct disorder: a descriptive analysis. J Evid Based Soc work 2014;11(4):350-9.

[27] Masi G, Milone A, Canepa G, Millepiedi S, Mucci M, Muratori F. Olanzapine treatment in adolescents with severe conduct disorder. Eur Psychiatry 2006;21(1):51-7.

[28] Teixeira EH, Celeri EV, Jacintho AC, Dalgalarrondo P. Clozapine in severe conduct disorder. J Child Adolesc Psychopharmacol 2013;23(1):44-8.

[29] Liu J, Raine A, Venables PH, Mednick SA. Malnutrition at age 3 years and externalizing behavior problems at ages 8, 11, and 17 years. Am J Psychiatry 2004;161(11):2005-13.

[30] Gesch B. Adolescence: Does good nutrition = good behaviour? Nutr Health 2013;22(1):55-65.

[31] Woodward TW. A review of the effects of martial arts practice on health. WMJ 2009;108(1):40-3.

Chapter 4

AGGRESSIVE BEHAVIORS

Joseph L Calles Jr.[*], MD

Department of Psychiatry, Western Michigan University Homer Stryker MD School of Medicine, Kalamazoo, Michigan, United States

Patients presenting with aggressive behaviors are commonly encountered in pediatric practice and are quite challenging to clinicians. The behaviors are usually manifestations of medical, substance-related and/or psychiatric disorders. This review will discuss aggression in terms of its definition, epidemiology, clinical features, various etiologies, and therapeutic interventions. Aggressive behaviors that present in pediatric care settings are symptoms of underlying medical, substance-related and/or psychiatric disorders. This review presents a clinical approach to the assessment of the subjective and objective features of aggression, as well as a guide to rational pharmaco-therapeutic interventions. It should be kept in mind that the use of psychotropic medications is but one part of the comprehensive management of aggression in children and adolescents.

INTRODUCTION

Aggression or behavior that is hostile, threatening and/or assaultive- has increasingly become a common clinical problem. Although aggression can be either verbal or physical, and the physical expression of aggression can be towards property or person, it is aggressive behavior directed towards people (i.e., violence) that generates the most concern from family members, school personnel, and the community at large. It also may cause a certain degree of discomfort for clinicians, as their backgrounds and training to help people runs counter to the described harmful and sometimes cruel behaviors perpetrated by some of their patients.

The pediatrician presented with an aggressive younger patient tends to ask two clinical questions: Why is this person behaving this way? How do I help this person? The purpose of this review is to guide the clinician in assessing the problem and initiating a rational treatment plan.

---

[*] Correspondence: Professor Joseph L. Calles Jr, Department of Psychiatry, Western Michigan University Homer Stryker MD School of Medicine, 1717 Shaffer Road, Suite 010, Kalamazoo, MI, 49048 United States. E-mail: joseph.calles@med.wmich.edu.

DEFINITION

We equate aggression with actions that are threatening or attacking, but there are also cognitive and affective components to the behaviors (see "Clinical Features" below). As we cannot know exactly what a person is thinking or feeling (unless he or she tells us), the clinical focus on the aggressive behaviors is important for two reasons. The first is that we can actually experience the other person's aggressive acts with our own senses, e.g., hearing verbalized threats or seeing assaultive acts. The second is that the people on the receiving end of the aggression are likely to be injured emotionally and/or physically.

Aggression is the end result of a process that begins with some type of provoking event- internal or external- that leads to overwhelming angry thoughts and/or feelings that are eventually expressed in words and/or actions (see figure 1).

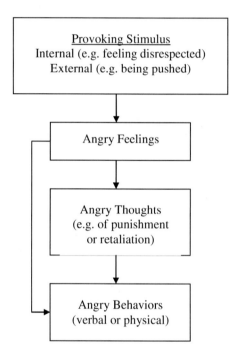

Figure 1.

The outward expression of anger, i.e., aggression, is usually conceptualized in terms of a hierarchy, with the least dangerous level being verbal, such as threats to harm someone (the old saying "sticks and stones may break my bones, but words will never harm me" comes to mind), and the most dangerous level being the harming of a person (see figure 2). In that regard, harming oneself is taken seriously, but harming someone else is taken even more seriously- as evidenced by the fact that most people who injure themselves come in contact with the healthcare system, whereas most people who injure others come in contact with the legal system. Multiple types of aggression will often be expressed simultaneously when people become extremely angry.

The sequence in figure 1 is not quite complete, in that aggression that starts with uncontrollable anger (as noted) can be called *reactive*, i.e., feelings override thinking. There is another type of aggression, called *proactive*, wherein thinking overrides (at least temporarily) feelings, i.e., the aggression can be delayed and planned for (often called "payback"). This chapter is only considering reactive aggression.

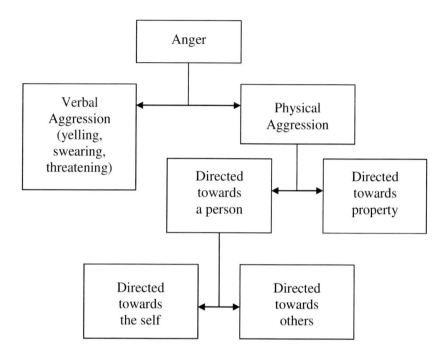

Figure 2.

EPIDEMIOLOGY

Every two years, the Centers for Disease Control and Prevention (CDC), of the U.S. Department of Health and Human Services, conduct their national Youth Risk Behavior Surveillance (YRBS) (1); the last complete data available cover September 2012-December 2013. In that survey, representative samples of public school students in grades 9-12 were carefully questioned about various risk behaviors.

Regarding those behaviors that have direct relevance to violence, the following statistics were reported for the 12 months preceding the survey: of all students, 24.7% had been in at least one fight, 3.1% had been in at least one fight that led to an injury that required medical intervention, 8.1% had been in at least one fight on school property, and 10.3% had experienced dating violence. In the *preceding 30 days*, of all students, on at least one occasion 17.9% had carried a weapon, 5.5% had carried a gun, and 5.2% had carried a weapon on school property. Also, during the 12 months before the survey, 6.9% of students had been threatened or injured with a weapon on school property. These data demonstrate that aggressive, violent, dangerous, and potentially lethal behaviors are- sadly- fairly common in the lives of American youth.

Informal surveys suggest that aggressive behaviors are presenting more commonly in pediatric care settings, straining resources and generating fear and frustration on the part of clinicians.

CLINICAL FEATURES

The presentation and course of aggression is quite variable, and depends on several factors:

- *Age of onset.* It appears that the use of aggression to deal with frustration, or to solve problems, is quite natural. By the age of 17 months most children display some physical aggression towards family members. It is the responsibility of the caregiving environment to model appropriate anger management. What happens when that guidance is lacking? Children who start out with high levels of aggression, which persists over time, are at greater risk of developing disruptive behavior disorders (2, 3). A minority of children (3%-7%) will develop high frequency physical aggression, a product of the interaction between genetic factors and early social experiences (5). That early-onset aggression is also more predictive of serious antisocial behavior into adulthood, even more so than are adolescent-onset aggressive behaviors (6).
- *Gender.* Before adolescence, boys consistently display more physical aggression than do girls; however, that is not to say that girls cannot be aggressive. Girls tend to engage in what is called *relational* aggression, which involves the use of criticism, negative rumors and social ostracism to hurt female peers. During adolescence there appears to be an increase in physical aggression in both males and females. In more recent years the rate of increase of serious aggressive acts (e.g., assaults) in adolescent females has been much greater than that seen in adolescent males (6); the cause is likely multifactorial in nature (7).
- *Intelligence.* In general, the lower a person's intellectual capability, the higher the risk for becoming aggressive. This probably derives from a combination of factors, including decreased/absent language skills, concrete thought processing, poor frustration tolerance, inability to delay gratification, and- depending on the nature of the intellectual impairment- the presence of seizure activity and psychiatric disorders.
- *Setting.* Some aggressive behaviors may be confined to specific locales, e.g., fighting only at school or being destructive only at home. In general, the more places that aggression is displayed, the more serious the problem.
- *Effects of media exposure.* Children- especially young ones- are impressionable. The playing of violent video games can desensitize children to the effects of violence, which in turn can increase the risk of using aggressive behavior as an inappropriate way to solve problems (8).
- *Context.* Aggression almost always derives from some type of interpersonal conflict (9). Its expression can be immediate (e.g., hitting someone after being pushed) or delayed (e.g., destroying a room at home following an argument at school). The quality and quantity of aggression can be modified by the social context within which it occurs. For example, peer pressure may influence a child to override his/her internal prohibition to fight. There is also a bidirectional relationship between

aggression and peer rejection, i.e., an increase in one increases the likelihood of the other. In general, the more impersonal the trigger of aggression the more serious the problem. A chilling example of this is a boy who seriously injured another boy- a stranger- just because he "didn't like the way he looks."

- *Cognitions.* What we tell ourselves is often more important than what others tell us, at least in regards to aggression. Making random eye contact with someone is usually unremarkable for most people. For people who have problems with anger dyscontrol, that act could be interpreted as a threat or a challenge, greatly increasing the probability that a verbal, or even physical, exchange will ensue. The aggression-prone individual is at high risk of perceiving the words and gestures of others as negative and personal; possible impressions are that the other person is being rude, disrespectful, or has "bad intentions" (10).
- *Affective state.* That there is a correlation between degree of anger and level of aggression seems fairly intuitive. Some people describe anger so intense that they "blackout," i.e., that they have little to no recall for their behavior, which can include serious property destruction or injury towards others (one adolescent male commented that, if people observing him hadn't pulled him off the other boy, "I probably would've killed him").
- *Past outcomes.* Every human event or situation has a behavioral element to it. Even in cases clearly involving psychiatrically-impaired individuals, how the environment (i.e., other people) responds to someone's aggressive behaviors will tend to either increase or decrease the probability of future episodes. An example is a family wherein their adolescent member assaults other members of the family and/or causes extensive property damage. Calling the police and filing criminal charges is likely to reduce the probability of similar future events. Conversely, having no negative consequences is likely to increase the odds of future episodes.
- *Degree of impulsivity.* Impulsivity- the tendency to act before thinking- is a risk factor for the reactive type of aggression. Some psychiatric conditions are associated with impulsivity and reactivity, and as such are risk factors for aggression (see "Diagnosis" below).
- *Degree of control.* The right amount of self-control can help an individual to avoid conflict, or to minimize it should it occur. People who are over-controlled may under-react to a conflictual situation. Depending on the other person's response style (i.e., impulsive vs. controlled), things may escalate in-part to try and elicit a reaction from the over-controlled individual. This may be part of the dynamic for a person who tends to be bullied, and who in turn is more likely to be a bully.
- *Parenting style.* In young children, how mothers parent can have an effect on the level of aggression displayed when children transgress against other children. At least one study has demonstrated that a parenting style with higher levels of maternal warmth and greater use of reasoning (i.e., an authoritative vs. authoritarian style) is associated with lower levels of child aggression (11). Conversely, lack of parental warmth and use of physical punishment are associated with oppositional behaviors and child aggression, respectively (12).

DIAGNOSIS

Aggression is not a diagnosis, but a symptom of a medical, substance-related and/or psychiatric disorder. Table 1 lists some of the more common conditions associated with aggressive behaviors.

Table 1. Disorders associated with aggressive behaviors

Medical
Seizure disorders
Sleep disorders
Traumatic brain injury
Encephalitis/meningitis
Sensory impairments
Developmental disorders:
• Fetal alcohol syndrome
• Fragile X syndrome
• Prader-Willi syndrome
• Angelman syndrome
• Tuberous sclerosis complex
• Smith-Magenis syndrome
• Cri du chat syndrome
Substance-related
Alcohol abuse/dependence: intoxication or withdrawal
Anxiolytic abuse/dependence: intoxication or withdrawal
Cannabis abuse/dependence: withdrawal
Stimulant abuse/dependence: intoxication
Psychiatric
Intellectual disabilities
Autism spectrum disorders
Speech-language disorders
Disruptive behavior disorders:
• Attention-deficit/hyperactivity disorder
• Oppositional defiant disorder
• Conduct disorder
Mood disorders:
• Major depressive disorder
• Disruptive mood dysregulation disorder
• Bipolar disorder
Anxiety disorders:
• Social anxiety disorder
• Separation anxiety disorder
Trauma-related disorders:
• Post-traumatic stress disorder
Schizophrenia and other psychotic disorders
Tic disorders
Intermittent explosive disorder
Personality disorders:
• Borderline personality disorder (mostly females)
• Antisocial personality disorder (mostly males; not diagnosed before age 18)
• Paranoid personality disorder (mostly males)

Medical disorders

The assessment of aggression begins with identifying medical problems that may be the source of irritability and anger that leads to aggressive behaviors; common conditions include:

- *Seizure disorders.* It has been appreciated for some time that seizure disorders can manifest as emotional disturbances, including aggressive behaviors. Much of the medical literature has focused on seizure foci in the temporal lobes, but reports of seizure-related aggression have also been related to epileptogenic activity in the frontal lobes and in benign epilepsy of childhood with centrotemporal spikes. It is the interictal period- not during the times immediately surrounding the seizures- when aggressive behaviors are likely to be displayed (13). Rarely, aggression may be associated with non-convulsive status epilepticus. An additional risk factor for aggression in those with seizure disorders is their high rate of psychiatric comorbidity, which itself increases the risk for aggressive behaviors (see "Psychiatric disorders" below).
- *Traumatic brain injury* (TBI). Non-fatal head injuries are over-represented in people under the age of 19 years, especially males. Serious neuropsychiatric sequelae of TBI- including aggression- are related to factors such as age (hyperactivity and aggressiveness increase as the children get older) (14), severity of injury, premorbid psychiatric status (e.g., the rate of *pre-injury* attention-deficit/hyperactivity disorder (ADHD) is quite high in TBI patients), and the development of seizures.
- *Encephalitis.* Infection-related inflammation of the brain has high morbidity and mortality associated with it. Especially problematic is encephalitis secondary to Herpes simplex virus (HSV), which has a predilection for the temporal lobes (15). As a result, post-HSV encephalitis patients, 50% of whom are children and young adults, can develop a myriad of neurobehavioral problems, including aggression (16). The psychiatric symptoms may be associated with seizure activity, which is a sequela of the encephalitis in almost one-half of the patients.
- *Sensory impairments.* Most of the literature on the presence of psychopathology in children with sensory impairments has focused on those with deafness, either as the primary sensory disorder or as part of multiple physical impairments. Internalizing disorders (e.g., anxiety or depression) are more common in deaf children than are externalizing disorders (e.g., conduct disorder), but both types are higher than in the hearing population, and the former may predispose to the latter. Aggressive behaviors in deaf children should be assumed to derive from factors *not* directly related to the deafness, except perhaps from the frustration associated with impaired communication ability (17).
- *Developmental disorders* (DDs). The practicing pediatrician will encounter children with a multitude of DDs, many of which will have behavioral disturbances- including aggression- as part of the clinical picture (18). Common DDs with high rates of aggressive behaviors (expressed towards self or others) are:
  – Fetal alcohol syndrome
  – Fragile X syndrome

- Prader-Willi syndrome
- Angelman syndrome
- Tuberous sclerosis complex
- Smith-Magenis syndrome

Substance-related disorders

The next step in the evaluation process is the ruling-out of drug and/or alcohol problems that may be provoking anger and aggression. The previously mentioned YRBS (from the CDC) found that, of all American high school students (males and females) surveyed, 70.8% had tried alcohol at least once in their lifetimes, 38.7% had recently used alcohol, and 21.9% had episodic heavy drinking. In the same survey, 39.9% had tried marijuana (cannabis) at least once in their lifetimes and 23.1% were current users. Finally, regarding stimulating drugs, 6.8% had lifetime and 3.0% had current cocaine use, and 3.8% had lifetime methamphetamine use (the figure for current use was not included). These numbers highlight the importance of exploring substance-use as a possible factor in aggressive behavior. The most common substance-use disorders associated with anger and aggression are:

- *Alcohol intoxication and withdrawal.* Some people who become intoxicated on alcohol can become angry and disinhibited, which can lead to assaultive and destructive behavior (the "mean drunk"). In those who develop alcohol dependence, withdrawal can include agitation and irritability, which can also lead to aggression, especially if their attempts to procure alcohol are thwarted (i.e., the person who tries to stop them becomes the target).
- *Anxiolytic intoxication and withdrawal.* The diversion of prescription anxiolytics and their availability to young people has increased over time. Although generally not as common- nor as severe- as alcohol-related problems, similar behaviors can be seen in younger people who are under the influence of, or withdrawing from, anxiolytic medications.
- *Cannabis (marijuana) withdrawal.* Agitation and aggression related to cannabis intoxication is uncommon. Its ability to calm someone makes its use attractive to those who are predisposed to anger and aggression, i.e., they tend to "self-medicate" with marijuana. A problem arises when the young person cannot obtain or otherwise use cannabis to calm themselves down, e.g., if they are getting drug tested while on probation. Cannabis withdrawal is better thought of as the recurrence of the underlying aggressive tendencies that the person has been suppressing with the cannabis use.
- *Stimulant intoxication.* Cocaine and methamphetamine (as well as other similar drugs) are powerful stimulants of the CNS. Depending on the amounts used, the social context, and the user's psychological makeup, stimulants may not promote euphoria or a sense of well-being, but instead may lead to irritability, anger, paranoia and hostility. The intoxicated person may respond to the negative emotional state with acts of aggression. Similar to the anxiolytics, prescription stimulants that are prescribed for ADHD are increasingly being diverted for recreational use.

Psychiatric disorders

The assessment of aggressive behaviors is completed by ruling-out psychiatric disorders (19) (see the other chapters in this book for guidance in the diagnosis and treatment of specific psychiatric conditions). The following disorders can include aggression as part of their symptom pictures:

- *Intellectual disabilities.* As mentioned previously, people with intellectual impairment are at higher risk for expressing negative emotional states as aggressive behavior. Although the lower the intelligence the more obvious the problem, younger people with mild mental retardation, borderline intellectual functioning, or even low normal intelligence may be missed, i.e., their cognitive limitations may not be appreciated. Experience has shown that intellectual testing is greatly under-employed in academic and clinical settings.
- *Autism spectrum disorders* (ASD). Younger people with ASD have difficulties in the areas of communication and socialization, and commonly also have intellectual difficulties. Due to their unusual behaviors, they may be targeted by other children, especially at school. The ensuing confusion and frustration may be expressed in any form of aggression, including self-injury. Higher functioning individuals with ASD may not be recognized as such when younger; fortunately, better public awareness is making this oversight less common.
- *Speech-language disorders.* There is a saying that "Those who don't talk, act." In those individuals for whom the ability to express themselves verbally is compromised, or absent, they are more likely to behaviorally act out negative emotional states, such as frustration or anger. The importance of developmental screening and early referral for speech-language evaluation cannot be overstated, especially in children with aggressive behaviors and delayed language milestones.
- *Disruptive behavior disorders.* This group includes ADHD, oppositional defiant disorder (ODD) and conduct disorder (CD). There is high overlap between ADHD and the other two disorders. They all have various degrees of physical impulsivity and emotional lability, poor frustration tolerance, and lack of awareness of- or concern for- how their behaviors affect those around them. In the case of ADHD, reactive aggression may play the key role through which hyperactive-impulsive behavior is associated with peer rejection (20). Given that those with ODD and CD come into conflict with authority figures, their aggressive behaviors not uncommonly lead to contact with the legal system, especially in the case of CD. Children and adolescents with ADHD, ODD and/or CD also have high rates of other psychiatric disorders, which must be ruled-out by the physician.
- *Mood disorders.* Aggression can predispose to the development of mood disorders, mood disorders can manifest as aggression, and mood disorders and aggression often coexist (21). Depression can be experienced by young people not only as sad, but also as mad. The anger and irritability can be so severe that aggression may not be limited to self-injury. The connection between depression and aggression seems to be more likely in youth who have lower levels of resilience in the face of environmental stressors (22). Depressed children and adolescents may get into fights with others or

may become destructive. At the other end of the mood spectrum, youngsters with bipolar disorder in the manic or hypomanic phase may not experience elation, but instead may be irritable, angry and aggressive.

- *Anxiety disorders.* Anxiety is an underappreciated, potential contributor to aggression (23). Children with *post-traumatic stress disorder* (PTSD) may act out recalled past traumas in aggressive ways. The trigger can be a nightmare, a re-living experience ("flashback"), or a reminder of the traumatic event(s) (e.g., people who look like the persons who hurt them). The aggression can look unprovoked or retaliatory, but is actually defensive in nature. Younger people with *social anxiety disorder* may become aggressive as a way of not going to, or getting out of, social situations that are too anxiety-provoking for them. Children with *separation anxiety disorder* may also fight to avoid being separated from the primary caregivers; conversely, they may attack- punish, if you will- the caregivers when reunited with them.
- *Psychotic disorders.* Psychosis in younger people is not very common; in fact, early-onset schizophrenia is rare. If psychosis is present, the affected youngster may become aggressive due to command hallucinations telling him/her to hurt people, or due to paranoid delusions that make the youngster feel threatened by others, or due to general mental disorganization and confusion that increases frustration and agitation.
- *Tic disorders.* Tourette disorder or syndrome (TS) is the prototypical tic disorder and has a high rate of psychiatric comorbidity, especially with ADHD, obsessive-compulsive disorder, and ODD. TS is also associated with episodic outbursts of anger and aggression called "rage attacks," which are not due to any specific etiology. They are usually sudden in onset, are very intense, can be violent, and may even be provoked by minor conflicts.
- *Intermittent explosive disorder* (IED). Similar to the aggressive outbursts of TS patients, the anger episodes of those with IED can be quite sudden reactions to even minimal provocation, can be quite severe and frightening, and can have serious consequences. This is a diagnosis of exclusion, as the symptoms should not be better accounted for by medical, substance-use or other psychiatric disorders. It is not uncommon for patients with IED to self-medicate with cannabis, which puts them at risk for increased aggression should they no longer be able to use the drug.
- *Disruptive mood dysregulation disorder* (DMDD). The DSM-5 has included this disorder (previously called severe mood dysregulation (SMD by some researchers), the hallmark of which is the presence of severe, recurrent temper tantrums, with an inter-episode mood that is persistently irritable or angry. The anger is commonly expressed as verbal rages or physical aggression towards people or property. This differs from bipolar disorder, which has normal mood (euthymia) in between episodes of depression and/or mania.
- *Personality disorders.* The Diagnostic and Statistical Manual, Fifth Edition (DSM-5), of American Psychiatric Association (24) allows for the diagnosis of personality disorders (except antisocial personality disorder) in those less than 18 years of age, providing that the clinical features have been "stable across time and consistent across situations," and are not due to another condition. The most common personality disorder encountered in child and adolescent psychiatry, that may manifest aggressive behaviors, is borderline personality disorder (BPD). Young

people with BPD tend to express aggression as self-injury, but they can also get into physical altercations with others (especially family members) and can be destructive (e.g., "trashing" their bedrooms). Since BPD in younger people can be comorbid with other psychiatric and substance-use disorders, the clinician should rule-out other etiologies before attributing the aggression to the BPD.

TREATMENT

Some general comments are in order before discussing the treatment of aggression associated with specific disorders. *Firstly*, as aggression is expressed behaviorally, intervention should include a plan based on a thorough behavioral assessment. *Secondly*, safety will be the primary consideration in the selection of a therapeutic intervention. A certain medication may seem like the logical first choice (e.g., an antidepressant for a depressed, angry child), but there may be a high likelihood of making the symptoms worse (e.g., if there are risk factors for bipolar disorder, the antidepressant could provoke the emergence of mania). *Thirdly*, in the presence of multiple disorders which may all be contributing to the aggression, the initial target for treatment should be the disorder that will have the worst prognosis if left untreated. *Fourthly*, unless the aggressive behaviors are so severe that rapid sedation is warranted (e.g., in an emergency department or inpatient unit), medications should be started singly, in low doses, and titrated slowly. The ideal goals should always be to avoid or minimize polypharmacy, and to use the lowest effective dosages (vs. always increasing dosages to "usual" or maximum amounts). *Lastly*, whenever possible and when available, treatments should follow evidence-based guidelines and algorithms.

Medical disorders

If the treatment of the medical condition is maximized and aggressive behaviors are still present, it is possible that there may be unidentified, comorbid psychiatric disorders that are the source of the aggression. Those should be sought out and treated.

- *Seizure disorders.* When there is clinical and EEG evidence that seizures have been controlled, the next step is to treat comorbid psychiatric disorders, such as depression, anxiety or psychosis. Psychotropic agents can be safely used in patients with seizure disorders, provided that dosing is done with caution (25).
- *Traumatic brain injury* (TBI). In the absence of seizure activity, the treatment of TBI-associated aggression can start with an alpha-2 agonist (clonidine or guanfacine) or a beta-blocker (propranolol or metoprolol). Pulse and blood pressure should be monitored closely. If not effective, anti-epileptic drugs (AED) or selective serotonin reuptake inhibitor (SSRI) antidepressants can be tried. Some groups have reported that the antiviral and anti-Parkinson drug amantadine can reduce agitation and aggression in post-TBI patients.
- *Encephalitis.* There is little in the medical literature to guide the use of psychotropic agents for aggressive behaviors related to encephalitis. However, given the

propensity for the HSV to affect the temporal lobes and create seizure foci, it is reasonable to use AEDs and avoid medications with the potential to lower the seizure threshold, especially the mood stabilizer lithium, the antipsychotic clozapine, and the antidepressant bupropion.

- *Sensory impairments.* In addition to treating psychiatric disorders in hearing-impaired children, it is very important that any communication deficits be addressed. Medications will not make up for a deaf child's inability to express his/her thoughts and feelings.
- *Developmental disorders* (DD). The pharmacologic treatment of aggression in DD is based on the presence of comorbid psychiatric and medical disorders. What follows are reasonable strategies for the use of psychotropic medications in select DD.
    - Fetal alcohol syndrome (FAS). Children and adolescents with FAS can have IED-like aggressive outbursts. As the prevalence of seizure disorders is not high in FAS, treatment can begin with lithium. If lithium is not effective, a trial of risperidone, an AED, or a beta-blocker should be considered.
    - Fragile X syndrome (FXS). Individuals with FXS can also present with symptoms of IED. Unlike in FAS, the incidence of seizure disorders is significant (15%-20%) in FXS. Therefore, treatment should begin with AED. If not effective, a beta-blocker, any atypical antipsychotic (AA) (except for clozapine), or lithium can be tried.
    - Prader-Willi syndrome (PWS). Children with PWS have a fair amount of anxiety and obsessive-compulsive features. Treatment may begin either with AED or SSRI. The next step would to use what was not tried initially. Finally, if the AED and SSRI are ineffective, buspirone or an AA may be used.
    - Angelman syndrome (AS). Epilepsy (chronic seizure disorders) are very common (80%-95%) in individuals with AS, with 50% developing seizures during their first year of life, and 75% developing seizures by 3 years of age. Therefore, a reasonable first step in the pharmacotherapy of aggression in patients with AS are the AEDs. However, seizures in AS are notoriously difficult to treat, and there are reports that seizures may be exacerbated by the use of carbamazepine, oxcarbazepine and vigabatrin (it's unknown if these agents may likewise exacerbate aggression). Sleep problems are also common in AS, which can contribute to irritability and aggressiveness. Melatonin (0.3-5.0 mg), before bedtime, is considered by many to be the treatment of choice.
    - Tuberous sclerosis complex (TSC). Patients with TSC also have high rates of seizure disorders (80% of patients). As in those with AS, the primary treatments for aggressive behaviors in those with TSC are the AEDs. There is also a significant rate of ADHD symptoms in those with TSC, so if the aggression is not responding to the AED, a trial of a stimulant or an alpha-2 agonist would be indicated.
    - Smith-Magenis syndrome (SMS). This disorder is also associated with high rates of seizure disorders (25%-50%) and ADHD symptoms. Treatment should begin with AED, followed by SSRI (as much of the aggression may be self-directed, possibly due to deficient serotonin). For prominent ADHD features either a

stimulant or an alpha-2 agonist may be used. Non-responsive cases may need to be treated with an AA.

Substance-related disorders

The primary intervention for young patients with drug and alcohol problems is formal substance abuse treatment, which usually involves individual, group, and family psychotherapy. If the substance abuse is secondary to another disorder, that problem should be identified and treated. If psychosocial interventions are not effective, patients may need to be evaluated for pharmacologic agents that may reduce drug/alcohol craving or the positive responses to the substances (see chapter 32).

Psychiatric disorders

When medical and substance-related disorders have been ruled-out, or adequately treated, the next task is to treat the psychiatric disorders that are causing or contributing to aggressive behaviors (26).

- *Intellectual disabilities.* There are no specific treatments for intellectual impairments or for the associated aggression. The AAs may be tried, with risperidone being a good first choice. If seizures are part of the clinical picture, then AEDs should be used first. The AEDs can also be used when the AAs are ineffective.
- *Autism spectrum disorders* (ASD). Risperidone and aripiprazole are approved for the treatment of irritability (and related aggression) in autistic disorder. If a seizure disorder is present (the prevalence of seizure disorders in autistic disorder is 20%-30%, and is correlated with intellectual level), then treatment should begin with an AED. Risperidone or aripiprazole may be used if seizures are well-controlled and irritability/aggression is not improved with AED therapy.
- *Speech-Language disorders.* Treatment is non-pharmacologic, and should be conducted by a qualified speech and language pathologist.
- *Disruptive behavior disorders.* For ODD and CD, the mainstay of treatment is a behavioral plan that consists of clearly defined, achievable goals and consistent consequences. If behavioral interventions are not working due to intense anger and aggressiveness, medications may have to be used. If other disorders are excluded or adequately treated, treatment with (in order) AAs, valproic acid, or lithium should be initiated. If those agents are ineffective, alpha-2 agonists or first-generation antipsychotics, such as chlorpromazine, may be tried (see Chapters 12 for details). For ADHD, treatment should begin with behavioral treatment and/or medication (27). The first-line medication should be a psychostimulant, such as methylphenidate (MPH) or mixed amphetamine salts (MAS) (28). Failure to respond to MPH and MAS should prompt a trial of an alpha-2 agonist or, in select cases, a beta-blocker (see Chapter 11 for details).

- *Mood disorders.* For the aggression associated with depression, the first choice is either fluoxetine or escitalopram, followed by another SSRI. In the event of SSRI failure, other types of antidepressants or lithium may be used. If bipolar depression is the cause of the aggressive behaviors, treatment choices are lithium, lamotrigine or quetiapine. If bipolar mania is the source of the aggression, treatment can begin with lithium, valproic acid, or any AA approved for use in bipolar mania (see Chapter 15 for details).
- *Anxiety disorders.* The agents of choice are the SSRI antidepressants. If they are ineffective, or if they worsen the aggression, then alternative choices are an alpha-2 agonist, buspirone, or gabapentin (see Chapter 16 for details).
- *Psychotic disorders.* One of the several available AAs should effectively treat psychosis and its associated aggressive behaviors. In the event that the AAs don't work, a first-generation antipsychotic (FGA), such as haloperidol, may be tried (see Chapter 30 for details).
- *Tic disorders.* In the case of TS, medication selection is based on which symptom cluster- the tic disorder itself, ADHD, or anxiety- is most prominent and most likely to be driving the aggressive behaviors. A safe first-choice that may positively affect all three clusters is an alpha-2 agonist. For unresponsive tics, an AA or haloperidol can be used. Unresponsive ADHD may be addressed with atomoxetine or a cautious trial of a stimulant. For persistent anxiety, SSRIs or buspirone are options.
- *Intermittent explosive disorder* (IED). The literature reports that SSRIs (especially fluoxetine) can be efficacious in the treatment of IED, and should be considered first-line agents, given their relative safety and ease of use. They should probably be avoided in patients with any features of a cyclic mood disorder. Other agents that have been used to treat IED (at least in adults) are phenytoin, oxcarbazepine (or carbamazepine), lamotrigine, topiramate, and lithium.
- *Disruptive mood dysregulation disorder* (DMDD). The literature in this area is scant. An open-label trial of risperidone produced a significant reduction in irritability in youth with SMD (29). In another study, the combination of methylphenidate and behavior modification reduced externalizing behaviors in subjects with combined SMD and ADHD. A randomized double-blind placebo-controlled trial of lithium did not demonstrate any significant effects on irritability and aggression when compared to placebo (30). Given its relationship to SMD, the treatment of DMDD should begin with risperidone, or another AA. If unresponsive, options would include the other agents used to treat mood disorders.
- *Personality disorders.* Patients with personality disorders can also suffer from other psychiatric conditions. However, pharmacotherapy will not alter the underlying pathologic character structure. Therefore, the treatment of personality disorders should be psychotherapeutic in nature, and should be carried out by a therapist experienced in working with younger people.

Table 2 summarizes the medication choices recommended for use in aggression associated with psychiatric disorders.

Table 2. Recommended pharmacotherapeutic agents

Disorder*	Medications** First choice	Second choice	Third choice
ADHD	MPH or MAS	Stimulant class not used as a 1st choice	Alpha-agonist or beta-blocker
Anxiety	SSRI	2nd SSRI or alpha2-agonist	Buspirone or gabapentin
ASD ± ID	Risperidone or aripiprazole	AA not used as a 1st choice	AED§
Bipolar disorder: -Depressed -Manic	- Lithium or LTG - Lithium	- LTG or lithium - VPA	- Quetiapine - AA
Conduct disorder	AA	VPA	Lithium
Depression	Fluoxetine or escitalopram	2nd SSRI	Non-SSRI AD or lithium
DMDD/SMD	Risperidone	2nd AA	3rd AA or mood stabilizer
DD: -FAS -FXS -PWS -AS -TSC -SMS	- Lithium - AED - SSRI or AED - AED† - AED - AED	- AED - AA or beta-blocker - AED or SSRI - 2nd AED† - 2nd AED - SSRI	- Risperidone or beta-blocker - Lithium - Buspirone or AA - 3rd AED† and/or melatonin - Stimulant or alpha2-agonist - Stimulant, alpha2-agonist, or AA
Encephalitis	AED	2nd AED	3rd AED
IED	SSRI	AED‡	Lithium
Psychosis	AA	2nd AA	3rd AA or FGA
TBI without seizures	Alpha-agonist or beta-blocker	AED or SSRI	SSRI or AED, possibly amantadine
TS; 1° symptoms: - tics - ADHD - anxiety	- Alpha-agonist - Alpha-agonist - Alpha-agonist	- AA - Atomoxetine - SSRI	- Haloperidol - Stimulant - Buspirone

* Abbreviations: ADHD = attention-deficit/hyperactivity disorder; AS = Angelman syndrome; ASD = autistic-spectrum disorder; DD = developmental disorders; DMDD = disruptive mood dysregulation disorder; FAS = fetal alcohol syndrome; FXS = fragile X syndrome; ID = intellectual disability; IED = intermittent explosive disorder; PWS = Prader-Willi syndrome; SMD = severe mood dysregulation; SMS = Smith-Magenis syndrome; TBI = traumatic brain injury; TS = Tourette syndrome; TSC = tuberous sclerosis complex.

** Abbreviations: AA = atypical antipsychotic; AD = antidepressant; AED = antiepileptic drug; FGA = first-generation antipsychotic; LTG = lamotrigine; MAS = mixed amphetamine salts; MPH = methylphenidate; SSRI = selective serotonin reuptake inhibitor; VPA = valproic acid.

§ = First choice if a seizure disorder is present.

† = Avoid use of **carbamazepine, oxcarbazepine and vigabatrin.**

‡ = In order of preference: **oxcarbazepine (or carbamazepine), lamotrigine, phenytoin and topiramate.**

Conclusion

Aggressive behaviors that present in pediatric care settings are symptoms of underlying medical, substance-related and/or psychiatric disorders. This review presents a clinical approach to the assessment of the subjective and objective features of aggression, as well as a guide to rational pharmacotherapeutic interventions. It should be kept in mind that the use of psychotropic medications is but one part of the comprehensive management of aggression in children and adolescents.

References

[1] Centers for Disease Control and Prevention. Youth Risk Behavior Surveillance- United States, 2013. MMWR 2014;63(SS 4):1-168.
[2] Hong JS, Tillman R, Luby JL. Disruptive behavior in preschool children: distinguishing normal misbehavior from markers of current and later childhood conduct disorder. J Pediatric 2015 Jan 8.
[3] Campbell SB, Spieker S, Burchinal M, Poe MD; the NICHD Early Child Care Research Network. Trajectories of aggression from toddlerhood to age 9 predict academic and social functioning through age 12. J Child Psychol Psychiatry 2006;47(8):791-800.
[4] Provençal N, Booij L, Tremblay RE. The developmental origins of chronic physical aggression: biological pathways triggered by early life adversity. J Exp Biol 2015;218(Pt 1):123-133.
[5] Asendorpf JB, Denissen JJA, van Aken MAG. Inhibited and aggressive preschool children at 23 years of age: Personality and social transitions into adulthood. Dev Psychol 2008;44(4):997-1011.
[6] Leschied AW, Cummings A, Van Brunschot M, Cunningham A, Saunders A. Female adolescent aggression: A review of the literature and the correlates of aggression, 2000-04. Ottawa: Public Works and Government Services Canada, JS4-1/2000-2E, 2000.
[7] Graves KN. Not always sugar and spice: Expanding theoretical and functional explanations for why females aggress. Aggress Violent Behav 2007;12(2):131-40.
[8] Brockmyer JF. Playing violent video games and desensitization to violence. Child Adolesc Psychiatr Clin N Am 2015;24(1):65-77.
[9] Cohen R, Hsueh Y, Russell KM, Ray GE. Beyond the individual: A consideration of context for the development of aggression. Aggress Violent Behav 2006;11:341-51.
[10] Cillessen AH, Lansu A, Van den Berg YH. Aggression, hostile attributions, status, and gender: a continued quest. Dev Psycholpathol 2014;26(3):635-44.
[11] Arsenio W, Ramos-Marcuse F. Children's moral emotions, narratives, and aggression: relations with maternal discipline and support. J Genet Psychol 2014;175(6):528-46.
[12] Stormshak EA, Bierman KL, McMahon RJ, Lengua LJ, Conduct Problems Prevention Research Group. Parenting practices and child disruptive behavior problems in early elementary school. J Clin Child Psychol 2000;29(1):17-29.
[13] Marsh L, Krauss GL. Aggression and violence in patients with epilepsy. Epilepsy Behav 2000;1: 160-8.
[14] Geraldina P, Mariarosaria L, Annarita A, Susanna G, Michela S, Alessandro D, Sandra S, Enrico C. Neuropsychiatric sequelae in TBI: a comparison across different age groups. Brain Inj 2003;17(10):835-46.
[15] Elbers JM, Bitnun A, Richardson SE, Ford-Jones EL, Tellier R, Wald RM, et al. A 12-year prospective study of childhood Herpes simplex encephalitis: Is there a broader spectrum of disease? Pediatrics 2007;119(2);e399-e407.
[16] Trimble MR, Mendez MF, Cummings JL. Neuropsychiatric symptoms from the temporolimbic lobes. J Neuropsychiatry Clin Neurosci 1997; 9(3):429-438.
[17] Roberts C, Hindley P. Practitioner review: The assessment and treatment of deaf children with psychiatric disorders. J Child Psychol Psychiatry 1999;40(2):151-65.

[18] Arron K, Oliver C, Moss J, Berg K, Burbidge C. The prevalence and phenomenology of self-injurious and aggressive behaviour in genetic syndromes. J Intellect Disabil Res 2011;55(2):109-20.
[19] Calles, JL Jr. Psychopharmacologic control of aggression and violence in children and adolescents. Pediatr Clin North Am 2011;58:73-84.
[20] Evans SC, Fite PJ, Hendrickson JL, Rubens SL, Mages AK. The role of reactive aggression in the link between hyperactive-impulsive behaviors and peer rejection in adolescents. Child Psychiatry Hum Dev 2015 Jan 1.
[21] Weisbrot DM, Ettinger AB. Aggression and violence in mood disorders. Child Adolesc Psychiatr Clin North Am 2002;11(3):649-71.
[22] Kassis W, Artz S, Scambor C, Scambor E, Moldenhauer S. Finding the way out: a non- dichotomous understanding of violence and depression resilience of adolescents who are exposed to family violence. Child Abuse Negl 2013;37 (2-3):181-99.
[23] Granic I. The role of anxiety in the development, maintenance, and treatment of childhood aggression. Dev Psychopathol 2014;26(4 Pt 2):1515-30.
[24] American Psychiatric Association. Diagnostic and Statistical Manual of Mental Disorders, 5th ed. Washington, DC: American Psychiatric Association, 2013.
[25] Gross A, Devinsky O, Westbrook LE, Wharton AH, Alper K. Psychotropic medication use in patients with epilepsy: effect on seizure frequency. J Neuropsychiatr Clin Neurosci 2000;12(4):458-64.
[26] Calles JL Jr, Nazeer A. Aggressive and violent behavior. In: Greydanus DE, Calles JL Jr, Patel DR, Nazeer A, Merrick J, eds. Clinical aspects of psychopharmacology in childhood and adolescence. Hauppauge, NY: Nova Science, 2011:103-14.
[27] Waxmonsky J, Pelham WE, Gnagy E, Cummings MR, O'Connor B, Majumdar A, et al. The efficacy and tolerability of methylphenidate and behavior modification in children with attention-deficit/hyperactivity disorder and severe mood dysregulation. J Child Adolesc Psychopharmacol 2008;18(6):573-88.
[28] Patel BD, Barzman DH. Pharmacology and pharmacogenetics of pediatric ADHD with associated aggression: a review. Psychiatr Q 2013;84(4):407-15.
[29] Krieger FV, Pheula GF, Coelho R, Zeni T, Tramontina S, Zeni CP, et al. An open-label trial of risperidone in children and adolescents with severe mood dysregulation. J Child Adolesc Psychopharmacol 2011;21(3):237-43.
[30] Dickstein DP, Towbin KE, Van Der Veen JW, Rich BA, Brotman MA, Knopf L, et al. Randomized double-blind placebo-controlled trial of lithium in youths with severe mood dysregulation. J Child Adolesc Psychopharmacol 2009;19(1):61-73.

Chapter 5

TWO DEPRESSIVE DISORDERS: MAJOR DEPRESSIVE AND DYSTHYMIC DISORDERS

Joseph L Calles Jr.[*], *MD*
Department of Psychiatry,
Western Michigan University Homer Stryker MD School of Medicine,
Kalamazoo, Michigan, United States

ABSTRACT

Children and adolescents with depressive disorders are commonly encountered in pediatric practice. These disorders cause subjective distress and functional impairment, and are often associated with other psychiatric disorders. Pediatricians are often in a position to first diagnose and treat depression in youth. It is important, therefore, that pediatric specialists learn to properly identify, fully assess, and effectively treat depression in their patients. The intent of this review was to provide information that will hopefully be useful in identifying and treating depression in younger patients. The clinician should be mindful of how depression may present at different developmental stages, the conditions that can mimic or co-exist with depression, and the potential adverse effects of antidepressant medications. Psychotherapy with cognitive-behavioral therapy (CBT) or interpersonal psychotherapy (IPT) should be utilized before pharmacotherapy for depression that is mild-to-moderate in degree, and should also be used as an adjunct to medication in the treatment of more severe depression.

INTRODUCTION

Throughout history, human beings have experienced low moods on a continuum, from ordinary *sadness*, to *dysphoria* (or depressed mood, the extreme end of normal sadness), to a *depressive syndrome* (characterized by a constellation of symptoms that we associate with depression, e.g., poor sleep, appetite, and energy), and, finally, to a *depressive disorder* (the

---

[*] Correspondence: Professor Joseph L Calles Jr, Department of Psychiatry, Western Michigan University Homer Stryker MD School of Medicine, 1717 Shaffer Road, Suite 010, Kalamazoo, MI 49048, United States. E-mail: joseph.calles@med.wmich.edu

requisite symptom cluster that also meets duration and impairment criteria). It is the depressive disorder that we refer to as the clinical state of depression. Our concepts of depression as a mental illness continue to evolve, as do the clinical criteria (the requisite symptoms and signs) which are currently incorporated into diagnostic systems such as the most recent edition (fifth) of the "Diagnostic and statistical manual of mental disorders" (DSM-5) (1).

DEFINITIONS

In this review only two depressive disorders will be discussed: major depressive disorder (MDD) and dysthymic disorder (DD), also known as persistent depressive disorder in DSM-5. The symptoms for the diagnosis of MDD in adults can be summarized in the well-known mnemonic "SIGECAPS" (see table 1). In children and adolescents, research to date has not found consistently significant deficits in cognition (including sustained attention and concentration) (2). Given that the clinical presentation of MDD is highly variable between individuals (at least 227 different symptom combinations can lead to the MDD diagnosis!), it has been difficult to identify more homogeneous subjects for genetic susceptibility studies (3). The symptoms of DD include similar disturbances of sleep, appetite, energy and concentration, with the additional symptoms of low self-esteem and hopelessness. For MDD the symptoms must be present nearly every day, during the same 2-week period, and represent a change from previous functioning.

Table 1. Criteria (SIGECAPS) for the diagnosis of MDD

At least five of the following symptoms during the same 2-week period*:
Sleep disturbance, either insomnia or hypersomnia
Interest in activities is diminished or absent**
Guilt, or other thoughts of self-blame or low self-worth
Energy is low and the person fatigues easily
Concentration is poor, thinking and decision-making impaired**
Appetite is poor and/or weight is lost (or not gained appropriately)
Psychomotor retardation or agitation***
Suicidal thoughts, plans, or attempts

* At least 1 symptom is either depressed mood or loss of interest/pleasure.
** Self-reported or observed by others *** Must be observed by others.

The DSM-5 does not specify unique diagnostic criteria for depression in children and adolescents. It has, however, modified the diagnostic criteria somewhat for younger patients, taking into consideration some developmental differences. For example, children or adolescents with either MDD or DD can have a mood that is irritable, rather than sad. Children with MDD may also not experience weight loss, but instead fail to make expected weight gains. For the diagnosis of DD in adults the duration of illness must be at least 2 years; for children and adolescents the duration must be at least 1 year.

EPIDEMIOLOGY

In recent years there has been a public perception of an "epidemic" of child and adolescent depression. Using concurrent assessments (vs. retrospective recall), over the last 30-plus years, no evidence was found for an increased prevalence (4). The reported incidence and prevalence data on child and adolescent depression have been highly variable, with several possible explanations for the differences. One factor is that different populations may have been studied, e.g., whether they were recruited from the community or from clinical settings. Another factor is the method of assessment; self-report questionnaires, general health surveys, and formal diagnostic interviews will elicit different types of psychological symptoms and yield different rates of depression.

Some examples are as follow (5):

- National Health Interview Survey (NHIS; 2007): Surveyed parents of 7,103 children and adolescents (ages 4-17 years). Of the total sample, 3.0% had received a diagnosis of depression during the previous 12 months;
- National Survey of Children's Health (NSCH; 2007): Surveyed parents of 78,042 children and adolescents (ages 3-17 years). Of the total sample, 3.9% had ever received a diagnosis of depression, and 2.1% had a current depression;
- National Survey on Drug Use and Health (NSDUH; 2010-11): Surveyed 45,500 adolescents (ages 12-17 years). Of the total sample, 12.8% had a lifetime history of a major depressive episode (MDE), and 8.1% reported an MDE during the previous 12 months;
- National Health and Nutrition Examination Survey (NHANES; 2007-10): Surveyed 1,782 adolescents (ages 12-17 years). Of the total sample, 6.7% reported a current (i.e. during the previous 2 weeks) depression.

In addition to the adolescents who experience a major depressive episode (MDE), there are increasing numbers of adolescents who report depressive symptoms that do not meet the full diagnostic criteria for an MDE, referred to as subthreshold depression (SD) (6). The point prevalence of SD is estimated to be 2.2% to 4.9% (ages 13-16 years), 12-month prevalence 5.25% t0 9.3% (ages 11-17 years), and lifetime prevalence 6.3% to 22.9% (ages 14-18 years). This is important information for clinicians to be aware of, since studies clearly show that adolescents with SD are at greater risk for developing a later MDE.

There is a difference between the genders as to when depression develops. Before puberty the rates of depression are roughly equal between males and females. Hormonal changes during puberty seem to be a significant contributing factor to the increase in depression in females (at least double the rate in males) (7). There are likely other, non-hormonal factors- including environmental ones- that also contribute to the increased risk during and after puberty. This is an especially important point to keep in mind, as external, non-biological issues (e.g., family dysfunction) need to be addressed for both the prevention and treatment of depression (see the section on "Treatment" below).

CLINICAL FEATURES

The signs and symptoms of depression can present differently at different ages, with much of the variability being related to developmental factors.

Depression in infants. An important feature of depression in this age group is *withdrawal*, the literal pulling away from the outside world (8). Depressed infants may stop responding to external stimuli, overreact to environmental stimulation, or display emotional distress with no apparent reason. They may also stop interacting with caregivers, e.g., avoiding eye contact or not reciprocating in social smiling. Attempts to console them by holding and cuddling may be met with indifference. The rhythms of normal biological functions- eating, sleeping, moving, etc. - become disturbed or never even get established. Appetite can decrease, and the infants will stop gaining weight, or actually lose weight. Sleep can be difficult to achieve or maintain, or can be excessive, but is always of poor quality. Motor activity is usually decreased, and the infant can appear listless or even catatonic. Previously acquired skills- such as crawling or speaking- may be lost.

Depressed infants may not necessarily display dramatic or obvious symptoms, especially early in the course of the illness (9). Vague or subtle changes may be missed or attributed to other reasons, which can delay diagnosis and treatment, placing the infant at risk for physical illness or even death.

Depression in preschoolers. Children in this age group with clinical depression can meet the usual DSM-IV-TR criteria for MDD, with modifications to account for developmental differences from adults (e.g., changing the duration of symptoms to less than 2 weeks, which is a very long time in the life of a preschooler). Aggressive play- such as with dolls or action figures- could reflect underlying themes of destruction or suicide. Sad or irritable mood in these young people is considered a *sensitivity* symptom, as essentially all depressed patients will endorse it; by comparison, anhedonia (the lack of interest or pleasure in usually enjoyed activities/possessions) is a *specificity* symptom, helping to differentiate depression from other types of psychopathology (10). Contrary to a previously held belief in so-called "masked depression," somatic symptoms are not a significant feature of depression in young children, although they may be a marker for an increased risk of developing depression.

Depression in school-age children. As children get older their verbal skills increase. One would, therefore, expect that depressed children would articulate their distress to those around them. In fact, depressed school-age children do report high levels of depressive symptoms when asked on screening questionnaires or during psychiatric interviews. Unfortunately, those same children tend to not report depression spontaneously, nor will they necessarily endorse depressive symptoms when asked by parents, teachers, or other adults in their lives. Parents and teachers will sometimes suspect that children in their charges are depressed. Teachers tend to have a higher level of suspicion (perhaps due to their experiences in working with large numbers of children) and are more likely than are parents to refer a depressed child for a formal evaluation. The school-age child who is depressed will often display similar signs of distress at home and at school. Social isolation and a preference to be alone manifest at home as staying in his/her room a lot, not eating with the family, etc.; at school there can be sitting apart in the lunchroom or avoidance of group play. Even in the absence of ADHD, depressed children- boys and girls- can appear restless and inattentive, with negative effects on academic functioning. The combination of irritability and disobedience commonly results in temper tantrums- usually outside of school- in both boys and girls. School-related behavioral problems are different between boys and girls, with the former more likely to get into fights, steal, and be destructive, the latter to be truant. Depressed boys are more likely to be bullied at school than to display bullying behavior, although at home they can intimidate family members with their threatening behaviors. Somatic symptoms in this age-group may be more common than seen in depressed preschoolers, but it may be an artifact of the high degree of comorbidity between depression and anxiety (see "Diagnosis" below). It is both interesting and of concern that, despite the previously mentioned symptoms, many teachers and parents- in the absence of somatic or behavioral symptoms- may miss the presence of depression in school-age children (11).

Depression in adolescents. Although boys and girls in this age group who are depressed are more likely to present with an adult-like picture of depression, there can be some important differences. One notable variation is in the reporting of the mood state itself: depressed adolescents may not actually feel *sad*, but rather irritable or angry, frustrated, bored, or numb (12, 13). Boys are more likely to experience a sense of restlessness, and tend to externalize their feelings, mostly with behaviors as verbal communication is diminished. They may attribute the cause of their suffering to people in the environment, especially parents. Girls are more likely to internalize their distress, feeling lonely, unattractive, and responsible for their misery.

Depression in college-age young adults. Symptoms of depression during adolescence may carry over into young adulthood, but may manifest more as functional impairments. In college students, there appears to be a bidirectional relationship between depression and academic performance; there also seems to be an inverse relationship between the two. Higher levels of depression are associated with poor grades, putting the depressed college student at risk of academic failure and early school withdrawal. The depressed young adult may also develop a substance-use disorder, which is more likely to exacerbate- not relieve- the dysphoric mood. The same impairments that contribute to poor school functioning may equally affect occupational performance in an adverse fashion. Finally, depression may lead to social isolation, which, alone or in combination with the other factors mentioned, increases the risk of the young adult committing suicide.

DIAGNOSIS

The presence of the previously described clinical features of depression should help the clinician to make the diagnosis of depression in a younger patient. There are, however, three issues that may jeopardize diagnostic accuracy: 1) medical conditions that may present as, or be comorbid with, depression; 2) substance use disorders that may cause or evolve from depression and 3) other neuropsychiatric disorders that can mimic or coexist with depression.

Medical disorders and depression. Patients in both general and specialty pediatric settings present with a myriad of medical disorders. Depending on the medical condition being treated, its severity and its chronicity, it is not uncommon for pediatric patients to complain of disturbed sleep and appetite, low energy, and difficulty concentrating. They may look psychomotor slowed. They may express feelings of sadness, helplessness and hopelessness. They may even wonder if life is worth living or wish for an end to their physical distress. On the surface this all sounds like depression, and it is obviously important not to miss diagnosing- and treating- it if it's there. It is equally important, however, to distinguish the depressive signs and symptoms that are concomitants of the *medical* disorder from those that may be indicative of a comorbid *psychiatric* disorder. The former should improve as the child is reassured and medical treatment proceeds; the latter may persist in the face of response to medical treatments, or may even interfere with successful treatment of the medical disorders.

Table 2. Medical conditions that may present with depression

Infectious
Mononucleosis (EBV or CMV)*
Influenza
Hepatitis
Human immunodeficiency virus (HIV)
Lyme disease (neuroborreliosis)
Neurologic
Epilepsy
Traumatic brain injury
Demyelinating diseases
Migraine headaches
Endocrine
Diabetes mellitus (Types 1 & 2)
Hypothyroidism
Hypercortisolism
Adrenal insufficiency
Exocrine
Cystic fibrosis
Hematologic
Iron deficiency anemia
Sickle cell anemia
Pulmonary
Asthma
Cardiac
Congenital anomalies
Cardiomyopathy
Post-transplantation
Renal
Chronic renal failure
Autoimmune
Rheumatoid arthritis
Systemic lupus erythematosus
Celiac disease
Gastrointestinal
Inflammatory bowel disease
Neoplastic
Leukemia
Lymphoma
Other
Chronic fatigue syndrome
Fibromyalgia
Other chronic pain syndromes

* EBV= Epstein-Barr virus; CMV= Cytomegalovirus.

A review of the medical literature found that depression was the most common affective prodrome of medical disorders (14). Diabetes mellitus (15) and epilepsy (16) are illnesses with higher rates of depression that require screening for depressive symptoms during regular office visits. Table 2 lists several medical disorders that may present with depression.

Substance use disorders (SUDS) and depression. A second group of disorders that can precede or follow depression are the substance use disorders (see table 3). The most common substances which have implications for effects on mood are:

- *Alcohol.* At least one-third of young people with both depression and alcohol abuse/dependence develop their depression after the onset of the alcohol problem (this is not surprising given that alcohol is a CNS depressant). An especial concern is that alcohol overuse can also be a risk factor for suicide.
- *Cannabis.* Another drug which can produce depression-like effects is cannabis, known more commonly as marijuana (MJ). Chronic users of MJ can develop what is known as an "amotivational syndrome." This is characterized by low energy and a lack of motivation, decreased concentration and memory, and a reduction or constriction of social relationships (associating mostly with other MJ users). At times the withdrawal from MJ can produce irritability, decreased appetite, and insomnia, which may be mistaken for depression.
- *Psychostimulants.* The use of CNS stimulants (especially cocaine and the amphetamines- prescription or illicit) initially causes feelings of exhilaration and well-being. As their use continues and increasing amounts produce less and less of a "kick," the positive emotional effects are replaced by feelings of irritability or numbness, low energy and motivation, poor concentration, and even suicidality- a picture indistinguishable from a clinical depression (which, if also present, is exacerbated during periods of withdrawal from the drug).
- *MDMA (3, 4-methylenedioxymethamphetamine).* Known as "Ecstasy" on the street, this drug, which is a modified methamphetamine, produces many of the same effects as the parent drug, including a depressive state (usually transient) upon withdrawal.

Other neuropsychiatric disorders and depression. Major depressive disorder in children and adolescents is highly comorbid with other psychiatric disorders, including the following:

Anxiety disorders. These are the most common co-occurring conditions in child and adolescent depression, with up to three-fourths of depressed youth having at least one anxiety disorder. The anxiety disorder will also precede the onset of depression- sometimes by years- in about two-thirds of cases (the exception is panic disorder, which tends to develop after the depression) (17). The combination of anxiety and depression is a risk factor for a more severe and longer lasting course of depression.

Dysthymic disorder (Persistent depressive disorder). At some point during the course of early onset DD (defined as starting before age 21 years) about 70%-80% of those who are suffering from it will also develop a MDD. Conversely, the presence of a MDD predisposes to the development of a DD, but at a lower rate (somewhere between 10% and 30%). Patients with this combination of "double depression" have more dysfunction, less competence, and a poorer prognosis than patients with either MDD or DD alone. The diagnosis of DD is likely to be missed due to a combination of its lower prevalence (vs. MDD) in the child population, less pronounced symptoms, and lower index of suspicion on the part of clinicians.

Table 3. Substance use disorders that may present with depression

Alcohol abuse or dependence
Amphetamine withdrawal
Cannabis abuse or dependence
Cocaine withdrawal
Hallucinogen abuse or dependence
Inhalant abuse or dependence
MDMA ("Ecstasy") withdrawal
Opioid dependence
Phencyclidine (PCP) abuse or dependence
Sedative/hypnotic/anxiolytic intoxication

Disruptive behavior disorders. Children and adolescents with conduct problems (i.e. oppositional defiant disorder [ODD] and/or conduct disorder [CD]) are at an increased risk for having a comorbid MDD, as are depressed youth at higher risk for developing disruptive behaviors (18). In clinical samples at least one-third of youth with MDD also have conduct problems, and more than one-half with conduct problems also meet criteria for MDD. Both ODD and CD are much more likely to develop after the MDD than before it, which speaks to the need for early diagnosis and treatment of the depression.

Attention deficit hyperactivity disorder (ADHD). ADHD also has high comorbidity with depression. It has been reported that 16%-26% of a school-aged, community sample with ADHD met criteria for a "depressive syndrome." In well-designed prevalence studies, rates of depression in the ADHD population were found to be between 9% and 38%, with the ADHD preceding the depression in the majority of cases.

Somatic symptom disorders. Children and adolescents with recurrent or chronic abdominal pain (CAP) are commonly seen in pediatric practice. In the majority of those cases there is an absence of demonstrable physical illness. It has been known for some time that there is a correlation between functional abdominal pain and depression (but a question as to which one causes the other). One guide to the diagnosis of depression in CAP is the presence of other, non-GI somatic symptoms. One study has suggested that the presence of 3 or more of the non-GI symptoms increases the sensitivity and specificity of identifying depression on more formal screening (19).

Neurodevelopmental disorders. The identification of depression in those with an intellectual and developmental disability (IDD) has been problematic. A more accurate diagnosis of depression in those with IDDs can be facilitated by relying less on subjective report (which is sometimes impossible to obtain in those with limited, or absent, verbal abilities) and more on objective observations- social withdrawal, sleep and appetite change, irritability, etc. - by caregivers and clinicians. In some of the IDDs (e.g., Down syndrome and velocardiofacial syndrome) the risk of depression increases with age; in others (e.g., fragile X syndrome) the degree of risk correlates with degree of intellectual impairment.

TREATMENT

There are three basic approaches to the treatment of depression in children and adolescents: 1) psychotherapy alone; 2) antidepressant (AD) medications alone and 3) the combination of medication and psychotherapy.

Psychotherapy. The indication for psychotherapy as the lone treatment for depression in younger patients is primarily based on the severity of the depression. In most cases of mild-to-moderate depression psychotherapy is the preferable first step. The type of psychotherapy is crucial, as cognitive-behavioral therapy (CBT) and interpersonal psychotherapy (IPT) have the best efficacy data behind them as treatments for child and adolescent depression. Impediments to this approach are the lack of competent CBT and/or IPT therapists (20, 21), inability to afford such therapy, and/or resistance by parents/guardians, who may want medications to be prescribed (expecting a "quick fix").

Medications. Although the prescribing of AD medication as the sole treatment for depression is common, it is usually not recommended, especially since its use may increase suicidal ideation in some patients (see "The 'black box' warning" below). Medication is also a poor substitute for psychotherapy, especially if psychological factors (such as low self-esteem or a pessimistic worldview) or environmental issues (such as a chaotic family life or poor peer relationships) are driving the depression. The use of AD medication would certainly be an important component in the treatment of depression that is more severe, is worsening, or is not responding to psychotherapy alone. Our knowledge about how ADs work in the treatment of depression is crude, as ongoing research is discovering that the pathogenesis of depression is much more complex than the "monoamine (serotonin) hypothesis" (22) would suggest (23).

The "black box" warning. Since 2004, the US Food and Drug Administration (FDA) have required that the manufacturers of AD medications place a "black box" (i.e. serious) warning in their prescribing information literature. The intent of the statement is to alert consumers and prescribers to the increased "risk of suicidal thinking and behavior (suicidality)" in children, adolescents, and young adults treated with ADs for MDD and "other psychiatric disorders." Although the risk for increased suicidality was small for both placebo and AD agents, the risk for the active agents was about two-times greater. Fortunately, in the clinical trials there were no completed suicides related to the use of AD agents.

Subsequent to the original FDA recommendations, re-analyses of data and ongoing research studies have yielded contradictory or inconclusive results regarding the relationship between the use of antidepressant medications and the risk of suicide in youth. An equally- if not more- important factor to keep in mind is that untreated depression has been shown to be consistently related to an increased risk of suicide.

Combined medication and psychotherapy. The Treatment for Adolescents with Depression Study (TADS) found that the treatment of depression with both AD medication and CBT offers some advantages over either treatment approach alone (24). Firstly, the combination accelerates improvement, i.e. patients respond more quickly and achieve functional improvement earlier. Secondly, the combination treatment that successfully treats the depression also reduces suicidal ideation and suicidal events. Lastly, that study also determined that when combining fluoxetine and CBT, 3 children would need to be treated for

1 to show much/very much improvement, whereas 50 children would need to be treated for 1 to display a harm-related event. This comparison yields a better likelihood of help-to-harm ratio (LHH) when compared to AD treatment alone.

This latter point should help to reassure parents about the use of ADs in their children (see "How to use antidepressant medications" below). The clinician should remember that the positive results from combined treatment were achieved in studies that used fluoxetine (25), which at the time was the only AD approved for the treatment of depression in younger patients. It is not known if- but may be reasonable to assume that- other ADs (which are effectively used as monotherapy) will also achieve similar results in combination with CBT.

How to use antidepressant medications. Once the decision is made to use AD medication, the next step is to choose a specific agent (26). In the US, only fluoxetine and escitalopram are approved for the treatment of MDD in children and adolescents (those ≥ 8-years of age for the former, ≥ 12-years of age for the latter), based on efficacy demonstrated in randomized, controlled studies (27). Most clinicians also use the other available antidepressants in routine practice. The use of paroxetine, however, is not recommended, as in randomized controlled trials (RCTs), it was no more effective than placebo in treating child and/or adolescent depression. The use of venlafaxine is also not recommended, since switching to it was no more effective than switching to a different SSRI in treatment-resistant, adolescent MDD, and it produced more adverse effects. Figure 1 shows one approach to the treatment of uncomplicated MDD in children and adolescents, and as can be seen either fluoxetine or escitalopram are the medications of choice at Level I (fluoxetine if the patient is below age 12 years). The agent not used at Level I, sertraline, or citalopram are reasonable alternatives at Level II, with selection dependent on tolerability and/or response to the other agents, patient and caregiver preferences, and affordability. For the depression associated with ADHD that is not improving with a stimulant, bupropion or duloxetine would be reasonable first-choices. Atomoxetine, which is used to treat ADHD, is a selective norepinephrine reuptake inhibitor, which theoretically should act as an antidepressant. In reality, however, it does not effectively treat depression in younger patients.

There are no ADs that are FDA-approved for the treatment of DD at any age; however, the same agents that are used for MDD can also be used for DD (28). The dosing guidelines for the ADs can be seen in Table 4. Although sometimes used to treat child and adolescent depression, most of the pediatric research on bupropion, venlafaxine and the MAOIs has been on ADHD, while most studies on duloxetine have been in the area of pain (see the respective chapters on ADHD and pain for details). Table 5 lists some common AD side effects, as well as some less common, but more serious, adverse effects.

Whether dosing the AD by milligrams per day, or milligrams per kilogram per day, the amount used should begin at the lower end of the range. This is especially important in younger children, in those that are at a low weight for age, in those with hepatic impairment, and/or in those on multiple other medications that may have adverse interactions with the AD.

Fluoxetine may be given once daily, as may the extended-release form of bupropion. The time of day chosen is usually the one that will best facilitate compliance, although mornings may be better, in that an evening AD medication may disrupt sleep in some patients.

The SSRIs sertraline, citalopram, and escitalopram are typically prescribed in adults as once-daily medications. In children and adolescents, however, a split dosage may be better, as the higher hepatic metabolism and renal clearance in younger people makes it nearly impossible to maintain effective 24-hour blood levels with once-daily dosing.

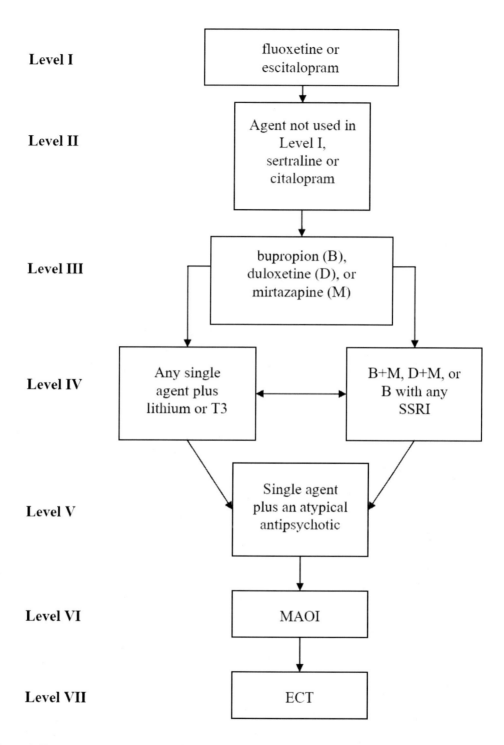

Figure 1. Treatment algorithm for uncomplicated MDD.

Table 4. Medications used for the treatment of depressive disorders

Class	Agent	Dosage ranges (daily)*
Antidepressants		
SSRIs	Fluoxetine	5-60 mg (0.25-1 mg/kg)
	Paroxetine[†]	5-40 mg (0.25-1 mg/kg)
	Sertraline	12.5-200 mg (1.5-3 mg/kg)
	Citalopram	5-40 mg
	Escitalopram	5-20 mg
SNRIs	Venlafaxine[†]	37.5-225 mg (1-3 mg/kg)
	Duloxetine	20-60 mg
Other	Trazodone	25-300 mg (2-5 mg/kg)
	Bupropion	75-300 mg (3-6 mg/kg)
	Mirtazapine	7.5-45 mg
MAOIs[†]	Isocarboxazid	5-40 mg
	Phenelzine	7.5-45 mg
	Tranylcypromine	5-30 mg
	Selegiline (transdermal)	6, 9, or 12 mg**

* Where dosing by weight is noted, the maximum daily dose should not exceed the upper limit of the dosage range for that respective medication, no matter the weight of the patient (given the high rates of overweight and obesity in the pediatric population).
** Each patch is effective for 24 hours.
† Generally not recommended for use in children and adolescents.

Table 5. Side effects associated with the use of antidepressant medications

Unwanted effects	SSRIs	SNRIs	Others
Common, mild-moderate:			
Agitation/irritability	X	X	X
Insomnia	X	X	X
Nausea, diarrhea, constipation	X	X	X
Change in appetite/weight	X	X	X
Dry mouth	X	X	X
Somnolence	X	X	M
Sweating	X	X	X
Headache	X	X	X
Dizziness	X	X	X
Infrequent-rare, moderate-severe:			
Akathisia	X	X	X
Hypertension/tachycardia	X	X	X
Serotonin syndrome	X	X	M
Abnormal bleeding	X	X	
Seizures	X	X	B
Hyponatremia	X	X	M
QT prolongation	X	X	
Acute narrow-angle glaucoma	X	X	
Bone fractures	X	X	
Hypercholesterolemia		X	M
Hepatic failure		D	
M= mirtazapine; B= bupropion; D= duloxetine			

As the risk for suicidality is highest early in the course of treatment with ADs (29), the FDA has suggested that patients be monitored face-to-face on a weekly basis during the first 4 weeks of treatment, then every other week for the next 4 weeks, then at 12 weeks, and as clinically indicated beyond that for the duration of treatment. The American Academy of Child and Adolescent Psychiatry has more reasonably suggested that monitoring be based on individual clinical needs and characteristics.

If the patient is not responding to the starting dose of medication, and if it is being tolerated, an increase in dose may be made after 2 weeks. Further dosage increases may be made every 2-4 weeks, depending on the degree of response and level of tolerance to the medication. If there is insufficient improvement in mood after 4-6 weeks at maximum dosage (or there are significant side effects at any dosage), the medication should be tapered off before starting another trial of AD medication.

If there has been insufficient progress at Level III (Figure 1), if the depression is worsening, or if suicidality is emerging, a referral should be made to a child and adolescent psychiatrist. Most pediatricians would likely not feel comfortable initiating treatments beyond Level III, unless they have had additional training in and/or experience with those modalities. This is especially true when considering augmentation with another medication, as there is insufficient study in that area regarding children and adolescents. Other concerns at or beyond Level III are:

- The addition of lithium at Level IV-A requires additional monitoring of hematologic, renal and thyroid parameters, as well as for the emergence of the serotonin syndrome if used with SSRIs, SNRIs, trazodone or mirtazapine;
- Level IV-B increases the risk of med-med interactions, including the serotonin syndrome;
- Level V requires additional monitoring of metabolic parameters, depending on the atypical antipsychotic selected (see the chapters on bipolar disorder and schizophrenia for details); and,
- Level VI requires close monitoring of diet and other medications used (including over-the-counter and herbal preparations) in order to avoid hypertensive crises.

Most depressed patients will fortunately respond to treatment well before Level IV. Some patients may seem to be "treatment refractory," i.e. they don't seem to be getting better, no matter what has been tried. Before proceeding to more controversial interventions, such as monoamine oxidase inhibitors (MAOIs) or electroconvulsive therapy (ECT), the following should be ruled-out:

- Insufficient dosing: It is quite common to see patients who have been given multiple medication trials, none of which have been titrated up to reasonable maximum dosages (some are so low as to be considered "homeopathic" in amount);
- Insufficient duration: This is often an artifact of impatience on the part of patient, parent and/or clinician. Switching ADs only after 1-2 weeks at the starting dose misses the opportunity to titrate up to a dose that may be effective;

- Lack of augmentation: Given the potential for serious side effects, some clinicians may not feel comfortable using lithium or atypical antipsychotics as adjunctive medications;
- Misdiagnosis: One thing to always consider is that it may not be "regular" depression, but actually the dysphoria associated with bipolar depression, schizoaffective disorder or schizophrenia;
- Comorbidity: As noted earlier in this chapter, comorbidity is common in younger patients with depression. Failure to identify and treat the comorbid disorder(s) makes it difficult- if not impossible- to successfully treat the depressive disorder.

In those rare instances in which ECT is necessary, that particular treatment will need to be carried out in one of the few academic centers that are qualified and authorized to perform the procedure.

CONCLUSION

The intent of this review was to provide information that will hopefully be useful in identifying and treating depression in younger patients. The clinician should be mindful of how depression may present at different developmental stages, the conditions that can mimic or co-exist with depression, and the potential adverse effects of antidepressant medications. Psychotherapy with CBT or IPT should be utilized before pharmacotherapy for depression that is mild-to-moderate in degree, and should also be used as an adjunct to medication in the treatment of more severe depression.

REFERENCES

[1] American Psychiatric Association. Diagnostic and statistical manual of mental disorders, 5th ed. Washington, DC: American Psychiatric Association, 2013.
[2] Vilgis V, Silk TJ, Vance A. Executive function and attention in children and adolescents with depressive disorders. Eur Child Adolesc Psychiatr 2015 Jan 30.
[3] Dunn EC, Brown RC, Dai Y, Rosand J, Nugent NR, Amstadter AB et al. Genetic determinants of depression: recent findings and future directions. Harv Rev Psychiatry 2015;23(1):1-18.
[4] Costello EJ, Erkanli A, Angold A. Is there an epidemic of child or adolescent depression? J
[5] Child Psychol Psychiatry 2006;47(12):1263-71.
[6] Centers for Disease Control and Prevention. Mental health surveillance among children- United States, 2005-2011. MMWR 2013;62(Suppl 2):1-35.
[7] Bertha EA, Balázs J. Subthreshold depression in adolescence: a systematic review. Eur Child Adolesc Psychiatry 2013 Apr 12. [Epub ahead of print]
[8] Angold A, Costello EJ. Puberty and depression. Child Adolesc Psychiatr Clin North Am 2006;15:919-37.
[9] Guedeney A. From early withdrawal reaction to infant depression: A baby alone does exist.
[10] Infant Ment Health J 1997;18(4):339-49.
[11] Keren M, Tyano S. Depression in infancy. Child Adolesc Psychiatr Clin North Am 2006;15:883-97.
[12] Luby JL, Heffelfinger AK, Mrakotsky C, Brown KM, Hessler MJ, Wallis JM, et al. The clinical picture of depression in preschool children. J Am Acad Child Adolesc Psychiatry
[13] 2003;42(3):340-8.

[14] Puura K, Almqvist F, Tamminen T, Piha J, Kumpulainen K, Räsänen E, et al. Children with symptoms of depression- What do the adults see? J Child Psychol Psychiatry 1998;39(4):577-85.
[15] Crowe M, Ward N, Dunnachie B, Roberts M. Characteristics of adolescent depression. Int J Ment Health Nursing 2006;15:10-8.
[16] Stringaris A, Zavos H, Leibenluft E, Maughan B, Eley TC. Adolescent irritability: phenotypic associations and genetic links with depressed mood. Am J Psychiatry 2012;169(1);47-54.
[17] Cosci F, Fava GA, Sonino N. Mood and anxiety disorders as early manifestations of medical illness: a systematic review. Psychother Psychosom 2015;84(1):22-9.
[18] Ducat L, Rubenstein A, Philipson LH, Anderson BJ. A review of the Mental Health Issues of Diabetes Conference. Diabetes Care 2015;38(2):333-338.
[19] Guilfoyle SM, Monahan S, Wesolowski C, Modi AC. Depression screening in pediatric epilepsy: evidence for the benefit of a behavioral medicine service in early detection. Epilepsy Behav 2015;44C:5-10.
[20] Avenevoli S, Stolar M, Li J, Dierker L, Ries Merikangas K. Comorbidity of depression in children and adolescents: models and evidence from a prospective high-risk family study.
[21] Biol Psychiatry 2001;49(12):1071-81.
[22] Wolff JC, Ollendick TH. The comorbidity of conduct problems and depression in childhood and adolescence. Clin Child Family Psychol Rev 2006;9(3/4):201-20.
[23] Little CA, Williams SE, Puzanovova M, Rudzinski ER, Walker LS. Multiple somatic symptoms linked to positive screen for depression in pediatric patients with chronic abdominal pain. J Pediatr Gastroenterol Nutr 2007;44(1):58-62.
[24] Sburlati ES, Schniering CA, Lyneham HJ, Rapee RM. A model of therapist competencies for the empirically supported cognitive behavioral treatment of child and adolescent anxiety and depressive disorders. Clin Child Fam Psychol Rev 2011;14(1):89-109.
[25] Sburlati ES, Lyneham HJ, Mufson LH, Schniering CA. A model of therapist competencies for the empirically supported interpersonal psychotherapy for adolescent depression. Clin Child Fam Psychol Rev 2012;15(2): 93-112.
[26] Pasquini M, Berardelli I, Biondi M. Ethiopathogenesis of depressive disorders. Clin Pract Epidemiol Ment Health 2014;10:166-71.
[27] Cai S, Huang S, Hao W. New hypothesis and treatment targets of depression: an integrated view of key findings. Neurosci Bull 2015;31(1):61-74.
[28] Maalouf FT, Brent DA. Child and adolescent depression intervention overview: what works, for whom and how well? Child Adolesc Psychiatr Clin North Am 2012;21(2):299-312.
[29] Baker K. Treatment and management of depression in children. Curr Paediatrics 2006;16:478-83.
[30] Picouto MD, Braquehais MD. Use of antidepressants for major depressive disorder in children and adolescents: clinical considerations. Int J Adolesc Med Health 2013;25(3):213-9.
[31] Sakolsky D, Birmaher B. Developmentally informed pharmacotherapy for child and adolescent depressive disorders. Child Adolesc Psychiatr Clin North Am 2012;21(2):313-25.
[32] Nobile M, Cataldo GM, Marino C, Molteni M. Diagnosis and treatment of dysthymia in children and adolescents. CNS Drugs 2003;17(13):927-46.
[33] Rey JM, Martin A. Selective serotonin reuptake inhibitors and suicidality in juveniles: review of the evidence and implications for clinical practice. Child Adolesc Psychiatr Clin North Am 2006;15:221-37.

In: Mental and Holistic Health: Some International Perspectives   ISBN: 978-1-63483-589-3
Editors: J. Calles Jr., D. Greydanus and J. Merrick   © 2015 Nova Science Publishers, Inc.

Chapter 6

CHRONIC ILLNESS:
PEDIATRIC BIPOLAR DISORDER

Amy E West, PhD and Mani N Pavuluri, MD, PhD*
Department of Psychiatry, University of Illinois at Chicago,
Chicago, Illinois, United States

ABSTRACT

Pediatric bipolar disorder (PBD) is a complex and multi-faceted disorder that demonstrates a unique clinical presentation and developmentally-specific symptoms compared to late adolescent or adult-onset bipolar disorder. Affect dysregulation is the central feature of this disorder and is associated with substantial psychosocial impairment. The primary goal of pharmacotherapy is mood stabilization, while including problem solving to deal with complex comorbid, residual, breakthrough and/or associated symptoms. It is imperative that any medication management be coupled with evidence-based psychosocial intervention that involves intensive parent and family work. In recent years there has been a tremendous increase in the number of children and adolescents diagnosed with bipolar disorder, some of whom may have been misdiagnosed and inappropriately treated. This review and the information contained herein should help clinicians improve the diagnostic accuracy of and treatment outcomes in bipolar disorder in younger patients.

INTRODUCTION

Pediatric bipolar disorder (PBD) is a chronic and debilitating illness that impairs children's emotional, cognitive, and social development. PBD is characterized by episodes of mood disturbance (e.g., fluctuating irritability/rage or elevated/expansive mood, and depression) and associated symptoms such as decreased need for sleep, grandiosity or inflated self-esteem, hypersexual behavior, racing thoughts, poor judgment, and impulsivity. These symptoms relate to significant impairments in social, academic, and family functioning (1, 2)

---

* Correspondence: Amy E West, Department of Psychiatry, University of Illinois at Chicago, 1747 W Roosevelt Road, MC 747, Chicago, IL 60608, United States. E-mail: awest@psych.uic.edu

and devastating long-term consequences including repeated hospitalizations and suicide attempts (3). PBD is recognized as a complex diagnosis and has been the focus of research and clinical debate for the past 20 years.

DEFINITION

Bipolar disorder has been classically characterized by mood states that fluctuate between the two "poles" of mania and depression, with periods of normal mood in between the episodes of extreme mood. PBD presents differently than adolescent- or adult-onset bipolar disorder; younger children with symptoms demonstrate longer episodes, more rapid cycling, and mixed mood states (4,5). Youth also present with considerable heterogeneity in their mood symptoms, and frequently experience symptoms of other disorders, such as attention deficit hyperactivity disorder (ADHD), oppositional defiant disorder (ODD), and anxiety disorders.

EPIDEMIOLOGY

Recent meta-analytic results suggest that PBD affects 1-2% of the population (6, 7). The accurate measurement of prevalence rates of PBD depends on the accurate diagnosis of PBD, which has been the focus of much debate. It relies on confirming mood episodes and accompanying symptoms, as listed above. Yet, this process becomes complex in the context of developmentally-specific symptom manifestation, overlapping symptoms with other disorders, and debate about how best to characterize mood symptoms in youth. In recent years, there has been increased discussion about how to distinguish authentic PBD from chronic mood dysregulation, in which youth experience non-episodic irritability and other mood symptoms. Chronic mood dysregulation has been targeted by those studying severe mood dysregulation (SMD) (8) and is the focus of the new DSM-5 diagnostic category of disruptive mood dysregulation disorder (DMDD) (9). Longitudinal studies will help clarify diagnostic boundaries for PBD by elucidating the neural underpinnings of chronic versus episodic mood dysregulation; however, PBD can be reliably diagnosed using DSM criteria (10, 11), demonstrates stability over time (12,13), and can be devastating for youth and their families.

CLINICAL FEATURES

PBD is still diagnosed using DSM-IV (and now DSM-5) (14, 15) criteria for adult bipolar disorder, despite debate over the clinical relevance of this practice. Children and adolescents must demonstrate recurrent periods of major depression and mania or hypomania fitting the classical definitions of BD type I or BD type II described in the DSM-5 (14). Developmentally-specific manifestations of core DSM bipolar symptoms in children are presented below.

- *Elated/expansive mood.* Patients are often excitable, silly, giddy, prone to uncontrolled laughter, feel invincible, and engage in excessive joking. They may describe feeling "overwhelmed" by their affect.
- *Irritable mood.* Patients present as easily irritated, aggressive, hostile, or acidic, with intense responses to affective stimuli that are out of proportion to what would be expected, and after which they are inconsolable. These responses may comprise aggressive behavior such as throwing things, slamming doors, difficulty transitioning, screaming, and kicking. Parents often report extreme rage episodes that are very disruptive to family life. Patients may feel remorse after and apologize for their behavior, using explanations such as "I tried to say no to my brain, but I can't stop feeling angry." Parents often tell clinicians that they "feel like they are walking on eggshells."
- *Symptoms of depression.* Patients may feel crabby, excessively whine, cry for no reason, look unhappy, spend hours in isolation, change moods rapidly from irritable to tearful, withdraw from friends and activities, engage in self-injurious behavior, or complain of somatic symptoms. These children often experience intense rejection sensitivity. Even young children may experience suicidal ideation and behavior, often stating a desire to stab or hang themselves. This likely represents a desperate attempt to regulate or escape from their intense mood swings. The rate of suicidal behavior in children with bipolar is high, with between one third and one half of children and adolescents with pediatric bipolar disorder (PBD) attempting suicide before they reach adulthood (16). Though psychotic depressive episodes are rare in younger children, mood-congruent delusions of doom, disaster, and nihilism are common.
- *Inflated self-esteem and grandiosity.* This symptom is characterized by statements such as "I am the best baseball player in America," "I will teach the coach how to swim, he doesn't have a clue," "I am absolutely sure that I am going to be the President," 'I am going to make millions on E-trade," with no evidence to support these statements. Delusions of grandiosity are differentiated from bragging if the age-appropriate reality check is absent and the child acts on the delusions.
- *Decreased need for sleep.* Parents describe their children as playing, singing, or watching television into the early morning, refusing to go to bed, and still not feeling tired in the morning. Children may use the description "I feel like an Energizer Bunny™."
- *Racing thoughts/pressured speech.* This state is often described by children as "My mind is going so fast, I can't stop it." Parents describe their children as constantly talking, never letting others have a say, being domineering, and constantly seeking attention by talking or "entertaining" excessively at home or school.
- *Constant goal-directed activity.* Patients are described as getting into everything and making a mess at home. Often, they get "stuck" on activities and cannot stop doing them. When confronted by parents, children will become defensive or deny responsibility. Clinically, parents often report their children are "always lying" and may describe "crazy maniacal spells." Parents may also report constant goal-directed behavior such as searching the web, playing chess, and washing the car all within a one-hour period.

- *Excessive pleasurable activities.* Children may have poor judgment and engage in excessive risk-taking behavior. They may call sexually-oriented chat lines, dress inappropriately, masturbate excessively, hoard and carry around pornographic pictures, simulate sexual activity with animals, use their parents' credit cards to pay for mail-ordered sex items, or pressure parents to buy expensive clothes or other items. Sexual abuse is often considered a differential diagnosis of these sexually uninhibited children.
- *Psychosis.* Patients can present with auditory or visual hallucinations, usually in addition to the mood-congruent delusions already described. Thought disorder can present as flight of ideas, becoming garbled if severe. Psychotic features vary according to the method of reporting and may be present in 17%-60% of PBD patients (17).

DIAGNOSIS

The accurate diagnosis of bipolar disorder is important to inform the application of appropriate and effective treatment. Diagnoses should be made by trained mental health professionals with experience and expertise in childhood mood disorders. In general, a bipolar spectrum disorder is diagnosed based on the presence of episodes of either extreme irritability or elevated, expansive mood in combination with other symptoms, including grandiosity, decreased need for sleep, hypersexuality, depressed mood, racing thoughts, and impulsive behavior. The diagnosis of PBD requires a careful assessment of the presence of discrete mood episodes and attention to the developmental manifestation of symptoms.

Youngstrom and colleagues (18) developed an evidence-based assessment protocol to increase the accuracy of PBD diagnosis, which involves (1) screening for mania, (2) establishing an actuarial estimate of the likelihood of PBD based on patient characteristics (e.g., family history of BD), (3) evaluating the diagnostic criteria with high specificity to PBD (e.g., decreased need for sleep, grandiosity), (4) obtaining clear evidence of episodes, and (5) extending the window of assessment to allow the clinician to observe mood fluctuations and assess symptoms over time. Screening for mania is one of the most important prognostic indicators for a bipolar diagnosis and can be used to preliminarily assess the presence of different types of mania symptoms. For example, the Child Mania Rating Scale-Parent version (CMRS-P) was designed and tested specifically to screen for PBD (19) and is a tool with excellent psychometric properties.

Bipolar I disorder is diagnosed if a child manifests clear symptoms of mania, such as abnormally elevated/expansive mood, grandiosity or inflated self-esteem, extreme irritability, hypersexuality (not explained by a history of sexual abuse), decreased need for sleep, and behavioral activation (characterized by agitation and pressured speech) coupled with poor judgment. Elevated mood, grandiosity, and irritability are the core symptoms of mania. Bipolar disorder type II tends to present with major depressive episodes alternating with hypomanic episodes. In these patients, depressive episodes dominate the clinical picture and cause major dysfunction.

It is often hard to characterize hypomania in youth, given developmentally appropriate excitability. Youth with bipolar disorder not otherwise specified (NOS) have fewer symptoms or symptoms of shorter duration than necessary to meet the full diagnosis. Because DSM criteria were designed to diagnose adult bipolar disorder and do not necessarily adequately capture the clinical presentation of BD in children, many youth with significant bipolar symptoms get characterized as BD NOS. This is primarily due to the fact that children tend to experience longer episodes with rapid cycling patterns and symptoms of mixed mood states compared to their adult counterparts (20). PBD symptoms tend to be chronic with superimposed episodes of more extreme symptoms; thus, discrete episodes can be difficult to discern and muddy the diagnostic picture. In addition, as stated previously, the diagnosis of PBD is further complicated by significant heterogeneity in symptom presentation and frequent co-occurring disorders such as attention deficit hyperactivity disorder (ADHD), oppositional defiant disorder (ODD), and anxiety disorders.

In the future, the diagnosis of PBD may be enhanced by a better understanding of the neurological underpinnings of observed symptoms and functional impairments. Children with PBD demonstrate cognitive impairments in learning, problem-solving, and cognitive/emotional modulation, including attention, working memory, executive function, verbal memory, and processing speed deficits relative to healthy controls and children with other disorders (21-27). These impairments have been shown to persist over time (28) and occurs independent of mood state (27). As brain imaging technology and other neuroscientific methods advance, this science may help reveal a neurobiological model of the complex interplay between brain circuits and feedback from the environment that can partially explain the pathogenesis of PBD and other disorders.

However, while diagnosis still relies entirely on report and observation of symptoms, it is critical to carefully monitor specific symptoms, the pattern of onset and offset of symptoms, and their developmental timeline. A comprehensive developmental history is important to understand the emergence of symptoms in context. For example, there is some evidence that PBD diagnosis may be preceded by a difficult temperament style in infancy and toddlerhood compared with children who do not develop PBD (29). ADHD and depression are also common precursors to a bipolar diagnosis. Indeed, most cases of pediatric bipolar disorder begin with a depressive episode (10,30), and up to 50% of youth initially diagnosed with depression go on to develop a bipolar spectrum disorder (31-33).

ADHD is typically diagnosed prior to PBD, but true comorbid ADHD should only be diagnosed if symptoms precede the onset of PBD symptoms or if the symptoms of ADHD are unresolved after successful treatment of the PBD. ADHD symptoms are highly co-occurring and it is possible that these symptoms represent residual symptoms of intrinsic over-activity and inattention observed in PBD. Family history of bipolar disorder adds value in considering the diagnosis (34). However, it is also important to note that family history should not be considered as a definitive diagnostic indicator. Conversely, the absence of a family history does not rule out the diagnosis of PBD.

Once a formal diagnosis of PBD is made through comprehensive psychiatric evaluation, additional evaluation should include: (1) the level of distress of the patient and the family, (2) knowledge, skills and attitude of parents, (3) school and social functioning, and (4) neurocognitive problems. These aspects of functioning may affect treatment engagement and participation, and would be appropriate targets for integrated pharmacological and psychosocial treatment.

TREATMENT

Pharmacotherapy. Based on the need to control acute symptoms, second generation antipsychotics (SGAs) appear to be the preferred first and immediate choice for pharmacological treatment of PBD. Aripiprazole (35), olanzapine (36), quetiapine (37), risperidone (38) and ziprasidone (39) are all viable FDA approved medications for pediatric mania.

In general, it appears that a combination of mood stabilizers is effective in the treatment of severe manic episodes of PBD (40-44), although further studies are needed (17). For example, the majority of these children need additional medications added to the primary mood stabilizer to treat concomitant symptoms such as attention-deficit, aggression, anxiety, psychosis, and sleep disturbance; however, results remain mixed in terms of the efficacy of additional medications to treat such co-occurring disorders (17). Pavuluri, et al. (45) integrated much of the available data to develop and test an evidence-based pharmacotherapy algorithm.

The basic principles of this algorithm model consist of the following components: 1) prescription hygiene; 2) mood stabilization; 3) overcoming the obstacles in mood stabilization by addressing break-through symptoms and 4) problem solving (for example, addressing treatment of comorbid conditions and/or adverse events of medications). The details are as follows:

- *Prescription hygiene.* In establishing a pharmacotherapeutic plan for mood stabilization, four things are important to consider. First, obtain a history of which medications worsened the patient's clinical status in the past, which were ineffective, and which were transiently useful or helpful. Second, rapidly wean off all ineffective medications. Third, discontinue selective serotonin reuptake inhibitors (SSRIs). Despite compelling data of SSRIs worsening or switching mania symptoms in the pediatric population (46), several children are still on substantial doses of SSRIs. PBD generally presents with mixed or dysphoric states, and many physicians tune into depressive symptoms and apply treatment at the cost of worsening the clinical state. Fourth, stimulants should be discontinued. Mood stabilization is the primary treatment objective and should be attained prior to controlling symptoms of ADHD. But, given the equivocal data (47-49) and the negative influence of stimulants (50-52), if parents report that they have been singularly helpful and showed a pattern of response independent of affect dysregulation, the practitioner may elect to continue stimulants at the lowest possible doses and preferably in long acting form.
- *Mood stabilization.* Currently there are several SGAs as well as lithium that have emerged as first choice medications in PBD. The SGAs alone may be effective when irritability is prominent and demands a faster response not possible with first-line mood stabilizers (45). Combination therapy of SGA plus lithium (or alternatively, lamotrigine, oxcarbazepine or divalproex) is an effective strategy as first-line treatment for severe cases, especially those with psychotic features (42,43). This strategy has the advantage of needing lower doses of SGAs compared to the doses potentially required for monotherapy, resulting in far less severe adverse events. While the practitioner excludes those medications that failed to be effective, he or

she can choose the next best option on the list either as an alternative monotherapeutic agent or for the combination regime (in severe cases or if monotherapy fails).

Table 1. Lithium and anti-epileptic mood stabilizer medications: Rationale behind the sequence for treatment of pediatric bipolar disorder (PBD)

Name	Pros	Cons
Lithium	• FDA-approved in children for acute mania and maintenance • Well-studied in adults • Works well in classic presentation	• Slow onset of action • Poor response to monotherapy • Frequent urination and hypothyroidism often cause concerns
Divalproex sodium	• Well studied in adult bipolar disorder • Effective when coupled with stimulants for comorbid ADHD	• Poor response to monotherapy in children • Poor tolerability: excitability, GI side effects, weight gain, sedation • Potential adverse effects on the liver and thrombocytopenia require regular laboratory monitoring
Carbamazepine	• Longstanding efficacy in adults	• Efficacy in children not established • Substantial side effect profile • Large number of drug interactions • Substantial laboratory monitoring required
Oxcarbazepine	• Anecdotal evidence suggesting that it may decrease aggression in PBD •	• Efficacy not established •
Lamotrigine	• Accruing evidence on maintenance for adult bipolar disorder • Considered as a primary choice, alongside lithium, for depression subtype • Potentially useful in combination with second generation antipsychotics, or lithium, for mixed or depressive episodes where depression is predominant	• Very slow titration over 6-8 weeks to avoid rash • Although serious rash is uncommon, benign rash, if it occurs, is treatable with prednisone and may limit ability to re-challenge
Topiramate	• May have some benefit in reducing weight •	• Negative trial in adult bipolar disorder • Cognitive dulling • Equivocal evidence available in PBD, including that for neutralizing weight gain as an adjuvant • Significant side effect profile

Table 2. Second generation antipsychotics (SGAs): Rationale behind the sequence for treatment of pediatric bipolar disorder (PBD)

Name*	Pros	Cons
Aripiprazole	• Emerging data on adult bipolar disorder and pediatric disorders	• EPS, nausea and vomiting • Response is not always predictable, with no knowledge on predictive factors
Risperidone	• Efficacy demonstrated in pediatric trials • It has a predictable response profile and reduces aggressive behavior	• Weight gain is common. • EPS and symptoms from prolactin elevation (e.g., menstrual disturbances) sometime affect tolerability
Quetiapine	• Efficacy demonstrated in pediatric trials • Little/no EPS	• Sedation and weight gain are common
Ziprasidone	• Weight neutral in pediatric studies	• EPS and less evidence for efficacy • Risk of prolonged QT interval requires cardiac monitoring
Olanzapine	• Good data in adult bipolar disorder and emerging data in PBD	• Severe weight gain limits tolerability and places children at risk for long-term sequelae
Clozapine	• Potentially useful in treatment resistant cases	• Mandated blood draws to check white blood count presents logistical challenges • Significant side effect profile often limits tolerability in children and puts them at risk for long-term sequelae

*With SGA use, one must consider the risk for metabolic syndrome (elevated lipids, high blood pressure and diabetes mellitus). Given that the level of such risk in children and the lifelong consequences of their use are unknown, these parameters require close monitoring.

Tables 1 and 2 summarize and provide a rationale for the sequence of medication choices by medication type. While these tables provide a basic guideline, the clinician needs to use his or her discretion in individual cases. In the development of this algorithm, levels of evidence dictated the order. General pros and cons of each medication are listed, as well as a rough estimate of relative efficacy. Some medications are better studied than others as a result of funding opportunities and the strategic plans set forth by drug companies. Other medications were considered as safe and effective based on studies in adult bipolar disorder. There is a paucity of head to head comparison trials that have been done in PBD. Furthermore, medications in these categories often take a long time to obtain pediatric indications. Therefore, it is difficult to make broad statements about efficacy comparisons (prescribing information for all medications are beyond the scope of this chapter) (53).

- *Addressing break-through symptoms.* PBD presents a multitude of clinical challenges beyond acute mood stabilization that must be factored into both the acute and maintenance phases of treatment, such as:
    o *Depression.* If there are prominent symptoms of depression, lithium or lamotrigine (54,55) are chosen as primary mood stabilizers either alone or as adjuvant to other partially effective agents. Second choice would be a

combination of lithium plus lamotrigine. Third choice is a small dose of SSRI (in desperate circumstances of severe depression). Any SSRI in small doses of 2.5 to 5 mg in a time-limited manner, under close supervision, and with psychoeducation is often effective alongside a mood stabilizer (56). It is important to balance the risks versus benefits given the black box warning associated with SSRI use in children.
- *Psychosis.* SGAs (if not on board already) must be added working down the list as indicated in Table 2 (45,57).
- *Persistent aggression.* The tactic in this context is switching to SGA monotherapy if mild aggression is present. In moderate to severe presentations, a combination of a mood stabilizer and an SGA is used, working down the list of choices (see Tables 1 and 2) after excluding ineffective medications and adequate trial of chosen medications. Clonidine can be used to subdue rage attacks when things are out of control (58,59). However, in our experience children can become disinhibited or become more aroused after persistent use, although this particular observation needs to be further examined.
- *Treatment resistance.* Chronic unremitting symptoms must be treated by using 1) alternative monotherapy, 2) at least two trials of combination regimes of mood stabilizers plus SGA, and then 3) moving on to triple therapy addressing comorbid conditions (for example, of additional stimulant for comorbid ADHD).
- *Sleep difficulties.* It is customary for the clinician to address sleep difficulties by increasing the PM dose of a sedating mood stabilizer. Beyond that, melatonin 1-3 mg (60) or trazodone 25-50 mg (61, 62) can be administered to establish a sleep routine, which is critical in managing PBD. While these compounds are not empirically supported by research in sleep intervention for PBD youth specifically, these compounds are known to be sedative, safe in the pediatric population, and interfere minimally with REM sleep. In subjects with abuse potential, benzodiazepines may be misused and medications such as trazodone may be effective alternatives (63).

- *Problem solving: Comorbid diagnoses and management*
  - *ADHD.* While ADHD is a distinct disorder separate from PBD, it is not understood if the ADHD-like symptoms in PBD warrant additional treatment beyond mood stabilization. In our study, several subjects continued to show symptoms of inattention post mood-stabilization that warranted stimulant medication (45). Cognitive difficulties such as shifting attention and impaired executive function seen in both ADHD and PBD can potentially be addressed by stimulants. Stimulants are almost always given in long acting form unless an additional after-school dose is required to sustain the benefits. Among psychostimulants, long-acting methylphenidate or mixed amphetamine salts are equally effective (64). Atomoxetine is factored into the algorithm as an alternative treatment if stimulants have been ineffective or not tolerated. There are no data establishing the safety or efficacy of atomoxetine in treating youth with co-morbid ADHD and PBD. Atomoxetine is a selective norepinephrine reuptake inhibitor with potential antidepressant effects and could theoretically trigger or exacerbate symptoms of mania in patients with PBD. Atomoxetine should be used with great care in youth with PBD.

- *Anxiety.* Anxiety disorders, including generalized anxiety disorder and separation anxiety disorder, are relatively common, especially in BD type I. Psychotherapeutic interventions, such as CBT, remain the first choice of treatment in children and adolescents with a co-morbid anxiety disorder. Small doses of SSRIs such as escitalopram XR as adjuvant medication may be effective if mania is stabilized, though there are no controlled trials for anxiety comorbid with bipolar disorder. SSRIs are the only medications consistently shown to be effective in controlled trials for childhood anxiety disorders (65-67). This treatment intervention requires educating the family about the risk of a manic switch, and close monitoring of the treatment response is necessary. Guanfacine may be considered if vigilance and autonomic hyperarousal are prominent (68). Benzodiazepines (69-71) and buspirone follow as alternative choices. Risk for developing dependence needs to be considered for long-term use of benzodiazepines in adolescents. Buspirone may not be effective in all cases. Propranolol may be considered in cases of performance anxiety. Medication is often utilized in small doses, to reduce risks of exacerbating bipolar disorder symptoms and to enable patients to benefit from psychotherapeutic interventions.
- *Problem solving: Management of selected common side-effects.* Low doses and slow titration are two fundamental principles that one may utilize to minimize the occurrence of treatment-emergent side-effects. If problems still continue, switching to an alternative medication may be necessary. For persistent side-effects in the context of a child who has responded well to treatment, consideration should be given to trying a lower dose of the medication prior to switching medications or employing pharmacological management strategies, as many side-effects are dose-related. When a risk-benefit analysis indicates that the offending drug needs to be retained at the desirable dose, strategies must be implemented to manage them. Some of the common challenges that require specific attention are listed below:
  - *Weight gain.* Despite several antidotes for weight loss, the single most important intervention is diet and exercise. If possible, consultation with a dietician is helpful. In our experience, simple weight management programs (e.g., Weight Watchers®) have been successful when followed along with a parent, but should only be done after consultation with a knowledgeable health professional. Timely meals and wise food choices help to cut down excessive calories. Weight gain from atypical antipsychotics and some antiepileptic agents often results from an increased appetite secondary to some pharmacological properties of these medications. Counseling parents that this may occur may help them to limit access to high calorie foods that may exacerbate this problem. Weight gain from lithium may partially be due to increased consumption of high calorie soft drinks or juice to compensate for the increased thirst caused by this medication. Limiting fluid intake to low calorie drinks is an easy way to prevent unnecessary weight gain.
  - *Extra pyramidal symptoms.* Benztropine 0.5-2 mg every other day to once a day is effective in combating extrapyramidal symptoms. Akathisia in patients treated with SGA is often missed and often responds to low doses of propranolol.

- *Sedation.* Night-time dosing decreases problems with sedation. In the event of residual morning somnolence, the evening dose may be moved to earlier in the evening.
- *Gastrointestinal (GI) symptoms.* GI upset from divalproex is dose related. Administering the medication with food and/or using a long acting preparation of divalproex sodium may decrease GI upset. Taking a SGA with a small snack 30 minutes to one hour before bed may decrease GI upset. GI upset from lithium is dose related and management strategy depends on whether the intolerance is specific to the upper or lower GI. Upper GI effects from lithium tend to be associated with high doses that directly irritate the stomach mucosa as well as high peak serum levels. Switching to a sustained release formulation or dividing doses BID-TID and/or administering the medication with food will reduce GI upset. Lower GI effects such as diarrhea are correlated with high doses and high serum levels. This also may occur secondary to residual lithium left in the large intestine, which may create an osmotic effect, drawing excess water into the lower GI, resulting in diarrhea. Lower GI effects may be managed by reducing the overall dose, switching from sustained release formulations to immediate release tablets/capsules or liquid formulations. Dividing high QD doses of immediate release formulations to BID-TID may also help.
- *Lithium related high thyroid stimulating hormone (TSH).* Elevations in thyroid stimulating hormone (TSH) occur in approximately 15% of patients. This usually occurs within the first four weeks of therapy and may normalize after transient elevation. Usually, new elevations are not evident after four years. In accordance with standard lithium monitoring guidelines, baseline monitoring of free T4 and TSH and then follow-up at one month, six months, then yearly until year four is recommended. Additional monitoring may be needed after substantial dose increases. If hyperthyroidism occurs and lithium needs to be continued, this may be effectively treated with levothyroxine titrated based on levels of TSH on follow up.

Since the commencement of our algorithm project and the subsequent publication of our feasibility study (45), we have continued to update our strategies and tactics based on new information. Aripiprazole is added to the list of SGAs. The role of lamotrigine has been elevated as specified in the scheme above. Atomoxetine was added as a second-line medication after trying stimulants for comorbid ADHD. In our experience, clonidine has been shown to cause worsening of symptoms in a subgroup of patients with PBD despite excellent short-term response for autonomic arousal. We are closely monitoring this phenomenon. Consequently, we are currently choosing guanfacine (given the longer half-life compared to clonidine) or propranolol as an alternative for extreme hyperarousal that does not respond to mood stabilization. Given the recent review presenting equivocal evidence of trazodone's efficacy as sleep medication (72), it was placed lower on the list after medications such as melatonin that had better data to support its safety and efficacy in idiopathic insomnia (60), although not tested for sleep problems directly in PBD.

Psychosocial therapies. While pharmacological treatment is often initiated immediately to control symptoms and stabilize mood, PBD is also associated with substantial psychosocial impairment across multiple life domains. Children with PBD demonstrate neurocognitive deficits and academic underperformance (25,73), disruptive behavior in school (74), and poor peer relationships and social skills deficits (56,75,76). In addition, family functioning is often wrought with frequent conflict (56,77), lower levels of warmth, family adaptability and cohesion (78,79), and chronic stress (80). Finally, youth with PBD often express low self-esteem, hopelessness, an external locus of control, and maladaptive coping strategies (81), all of which complicate treatment outcome and optimal psychosocial functioning.

There are several evidence-based psychosocial interventions designed for adjunctive use with pharmacotherapy to target PBD symptoms and functioning. The scientific foundation for psychosocial treatments in PBD has advanced significantly in the past ten years, yet randomized controlled trials are still limited. For younger children, child- and family-focused cognitive-behavioral treatment (CFF-CBT) and multi-family/individual psycho-education (MFPG/IFP) have been developed and studied. For adolescents, several evidence-based adult treatments have been adapted, including family-focused treatment (FFT), dialectical behavioral treatment (DBT), and interpersonal and social rhythm therapy (IPSRT).

CFF-CBT is a family-focused psychosocial intervention developed for children ages 7-13 with bipolar spectrum disorders and their families (82). This intervention integrates cognitive-behavioral approaches with psycho-education, interpersonal psychotherapy, mindfulness, and positive psychology techniques, and is employed across multiple domains, including individual, family, peer, and school. CFF-CBT is a manual-based treatment and is delivered across 12 weekly sessions, most of which are parent and/or family sessions. Key components of CFF-CBT are captured by the acronym RAINBOW (it is also called RAINBOW treatment): **R**outine, **A**ffect regulation, **I** can do it (self-efficacy boosting), **N**o negative thoughts and live in the now (CBT and mindfulness), **B**e a good friend and balanced lifestyle for parents, **O**h, how do we solve this problem, and **W**ays to find social support. Specific interventions include establishing a predictable routine, regular mood monitoring, teaching behavioral management, increasing parent and child self-efficacy, decreasing negative cognitions, improving social functioning, engaging in collaborative problem-solving, and increasing social support. Preliminary studies support the feasibility, acceptability, and efficacy of CFF-CBT in individual (83), group (2), and maintenance models (84). A randomized clinical trial was recently completed and findings suggest that CFF-CBT results in significantly greater improvements in symptoms of mania and depression, and global psychosocial functioning as compared to the control psychosocial treatment-as-usual (85).

A psychoeducational intervention, also aimed at younger children (8-12) with either PBD or depression, was developed by Fristad and colleagues (86,87). This intervention was originally developed in a multi-family group format (MFPG), delivered across eight sessions, and focused on teaching parents and children about the child's illness, treatment approaches, symptom management, problem-solving and communication skills, coping skills, and providing support for the parents. Randomized clinical trial results indicated that MFPG reduced mood symptoms (87). MFPG has now been adapted into an individual format (IFP) delivered across 24 sessions, which has demonstrated efficacy in a small randomized controlled trial (88).

Miklowitz and colleagues (89) adapted their family-focused treatment (FFT) for adults with bipolar disorder for use with adolescents (FFT-A). The goal of FFT-A is to reduce mood symptoms and increase functioning by facilitating an increased understanding of the bipolar disorder and coping skills, decreasing conflict in the family system, and improving family communication and problem-solving. FFT-A is a manual-based treatment delivered across 21 individual family sessions over the course of nine months; the content is organized into three core components – psycho-education (e.g., understanding the etiology and course of the disorder), communication enhancement training (e.g., role playing how to ask for help and use effective listening skills), and problem solving (e.g., identifying problems and generating solutions). Randomized clinical trial data indicated that FFT-A was associated with a shorter time to recovery, less time in depressive episodes, and lower depression severity scores for two years (90).

Goldstein and colleagues have adapted dialectical behavioral therapy (DBT)—originally developed for adults with borderline personality traits—to adolescents with bipolar disorder (91). DBT for adolescents with bipolar disorder is delivered over the course of one year, and involves two core modalities: family skills training (delivered to the whole family) and individual psychotherapy for the adolescent. The acute treatment phase is six months of 24 weekly sessions that alternate between individual and family therapy, then 12 additional sessions tapering in frequency over the rest of the year. A small, preliminary open trial of DBT in 10 adolescents with bipolar disorder demonstrated decreases in suicidality, non-suicidal self-injurious behavior, emotional dysregulation, and depression symptoms after the intervention (91).

Finally, Hlastala and colleagues have adapted interpersonal and social rhythm therapy for adolescents (IPSRT-A) with bipolar disorder (92). IPSRT is a psychotherapy program for adults with bipolar disorder that focuses on instability of circadian rhythms and neurotransmitter systems as the key point of intervention. Interventions aim to stabilize sleep and social routines, and address interpersonal triggers for mood dysregulation such as interpersonal conflict, role transitions, and interpersonal functioning deficits. IPSRT is primarily an individual treatment, but this version does incorporate brief family psychotherapy. A pilot study of IPSRT-A indicated decreased symptoms and improved social functioning from pre- to post-treatment (93).

CONCLUSION

PBD is a complex and multi-faceted disorder that demonstrates a unique clinical presentation and developmentally-specific symptoms compared to late adolescent or adult-onset bipolar disorder. Affect dysregulation is the central feature of this disorder and is associated with substantial psychosocial impairment. The primary goal of pharmacotherapy is mood stabilization while including problem solving to deal with complex comorbid, residual, breakthrough and/or associated symptoms. It is imperative that any medication management be coupled with evidence-based psychosocial intervention that involves intensive parent and family work.

REFERENCES

[1] Goldstein TR, Birmaher B, Axelson D, Goldstein BI, Gill MK, Esposito-Smythers C, et al. Family environment and suicidal ideation among bipolar youth. Arch Suicide Res 2009;13(4):378-88.

[2] West AE, Pavuluri MN. Psychosocial treatments for childhood and adolescent bipolar disorder. Child Adolesc Psychiatr Clin North Am 2009;18(2):471-82, x-xi.

[3] Lewinsohn PM, Klein DN, Seeley JR. Bipolar disorders in a community sample of older adolescents: prevalence, phenomenology, comorbidity, and course. J Am Acad Child Adolesc Psychiatry 1995;34(4):454-63.

[4] Findling RL, Gracious BL, McNamara NK, Youngstrom EA, Demeter CA, Branicky LA, et al. Rapid, continuous cycling and psychiatric co-morbidity in pediatric bipolar I disorder. Bipolar Disord 2001;3(4):202-10.

[5] Axelson D, Birmaher B, Strober M, Gill MK, Valeri S, Chiappetta L, et al. Phenomenology of children and adolescents with bipolar spectrum disorders. Arch Gen Psychiatry 2006;63(10):1139-48.

[6] Merikangas KR, Tohen M. Epidemiology of bipolar disorder in adults and children. In: Tsuang MT, Tohen M, Jones PB, eds. Textbook in psychiatric epidemiology, Third ed. New York: John Wiley, 2011:329-42.

[7] Van Meter AR, Moreira AL, Youngstrom EA. Meta-analysis of epidemiologic studies of pediatric bipolar disorder. J Clin Psychiatry 2011;72(9):1250-6.

[8] Brotman MA, Schmajuk M, Rich BA, Dickstein DP, Guyer AE, Costello EJ, et al. Prevalence, clinical correlates, and longitudinal course of severe mood dysregulation in children. Biol Psychiatry 2006;60(9):991-7.

[9] Axelson D, Findling RL, Fristad MA, Kowatch RA, Youngstrom EA, Horwitz SM, et al. Examining the proposed disruptive mood dysregulation disorder diagnosis in children in the Longitudinal Assessment of Manic Symptoms study. J Clin Psychiatry 2012;73(10):1342-50.

[10] Birmaher B, Axelson D, Goldstein B, Strober M, Gill MK, Hunt J, et al. Four-year longitudinal course of children and adolescents with bipolar spectrum disorders: the Course and Outcome of Bipolar Youth (COBY) study. Am J Psychiatry 2009;166(7):795-804.

[11] Youngstrom EA, Birmaher B, Findling RL. Pediatric bipolar disorder: validity, phenomenology, and recommendations for diagnosis. Bipolar Disord 2008;10(1 Pt 2):194-214.

[12] Geller B, Craney JL, Bolhofner K, DelBello MP, Williams M, Zimerman B. One-year recovery and relapse rates of children with a prepubertal and early adolescent bipolar disorder phenotype. Am J Psychiatry 2001;158(2):303-5.

[13] Geller B, Tillman R, Bolhofner K, Zimerman B. Child bipolar I disorder: prospective continuity with adult bipolar I disorder; characteristics of second and third episodes; predictors of 8-year outcome. Arch Gen Psychiatry 2008;65(10):1125-33.

[14] American Psychiatric Association. (2013). *Diagnostic and statistical manual of mental disorders* (5th ed.). Washington, DC:

[15] Diagnostic and statistical manual of mental disorders, 5th edition. Washington, DC: American Psychiatric Association, 2013.

[16] Lewinsohn PM, Seeley JR, Klein DN. Bipolar disorder in adolescents: epidemiology and suicidal behavior. In: Geller B, DelBello M, eds. Bipolar disorder in childhood and early adolescence. New York: Guilford, 2003:7-24.

[17] Pavuluri MN, Birmaher B, Naylor MW. Pediatric bipolar disorder: a review of the past 10 years. J Am Acad Child Adolesc Psychiatry 2005;44(9):846-71.

[18] Youngstrom EA, Findling RL, Youngstrom JK, Calabrese JR. Toward an evidence-based assessment of pediatric bipolar disorder. J Clin Child Adolesc Psychol 2005;34(3):433-48.

[19] Pavuluri MN, Henry DB, Devineni B, Carbray JA, Birmaher B. Child mania rating scale: development, reliability, and validity. J Am Acad Child Adolesc Psychiatry 2006;45(5):550-60.

[20] Leibenluft E, Charney DS, Towbin KE, Bhangoo RK, Pine DS. Defining clinical phenotypes of juvenile mania. Am J Psychiatry 2003;160(3):430-7.

[21] Bearden CE, Glahn DC, Monkul ES, Barrett J, Najt P, Kaur S, et al. Sources of declarative memory impairment in bipolar disorder: mnemonic processes and clinical features. J Psychiatr Res 2006;40(1):47-58.

[22] Dickstein DP, Nelson EE, McClure EB, Grimley ME, Knopf L, Brotman MA, et al. Cognitive flexibility in phenotypes of pediatric bipolar disorder. J Am Acad Child Adolesc Psychiatry 2007;46(3):341-55.

[23] Dickstein DP, Treland JE, Snow J, McClure EB, Mehta MS, Towbin KE, et al. Neuropsychological performance in pediatric bipolar disorder. Biol Psychiatry 2004;55(1):32-9.

[24] Doyle AE, Wilens TE, Kwon A, Seidman LJ, Faraone SV, Fried R, et al. Neuropsychological functioning in youth with bipolar disorder. Biol Psychiatry 2005;58(7):540-8.
[25] Henin A, Mick E, Biederman J, Fried R, Wozniak J, Faraone SV, et al. Can bipolar disorder-specific neuropsychological impairments in children be identified? J Consult Clin Psychol 2007;75(2):210-20.
[26] McClure EB, Treland JE, Snow J, Dickstein DP, Towbin KE, Charney DS, et al. Memory and learning in pediatric bipolar disorder. J Am Acad Child Adolesc Psychiatry 2005;44(5):461-9.
[27] Pavuluri MN, Schenkel LS, Aryal S, Harral EM, Hill SK, Herbener ES, et al. Neurocognitive function in unmedicated manic and medicated euthymic pediatric bipolar patients. Am J Psychiatry 2006;163(2):286-93.
[28] Pavuluri MN, West A, Hill SK, Jindal K, Sweeney JA. Neurocognitive function in pediatric bipolar disorder: 3-year follow-up shows cognitive development lagging behind healthy youths. J Am Acad Child Adolesc Psychiatry 2009;48(3):299-307.
[29] West AE, Schenkel LS, Pavuluri MN. Early childhood temperament in pediatric bipolar disorder and attention deficit hyperactivity disorder. J Clin Psychol 2008;64(4):402-21.
[30] Birmaher B, Axelson D, Strober M, Gill MK, Valeri S, Chiappetta L, et al. Clinical course of children and adolescents with bipolar spectrum disorders. Arch Gen Psychiatry 2006;63(2):175-83.
[31] Cosgrove VE, Roybal D, Chang KD. Bipolar depression in pediatric populations : epidemiology and management. Paediatr Drugs 2013;15(2):83-91.
[32] Geller B, Zimerman B, Williams M, Bolhofner K, Craney JL. Bipolar disorder at prospective follow-up of adults who had prepubertal major depressive disorder. Am J Psychiatry 2001;158(1):125-7.
[33] Strober M, Lampert C, Schmidt S, Morrell W. The course of major depressive disorder in adolescents: I. Recovery and risk of manic switching in a follow-up of psychotic and nonpsychotic subtypes. J Am Acad Child Adolesc Psychiatry 1993;32(1):34-42.
[34] Faraone SV, Glatt SJ, Tsuang MT. The genetics of pediatric-onset bipolar disorder. Biol Psychiatry 2003;53(11):970-7.
[35] Findling RL, Nyilas M, Forbes RA, McQuade RD, Jin N, Iwamoto T, et al. Acute treatment of pediatric bipolar I disorder, manic or mixed episode, with aripiprazole: a randomized, double-blind, placebo-controlled study. J Clin Psychiatry 2009;70(10):1441-51.
[36] Tohen M, Kryzhanovskaya L, Carlson G, Delbello M, Wozniak J, Kowatch R, et al. Olanzapine versus placebo in the treatment of adolescents with bipolar mania. Am J Psychiatry 2007;164(10):1547-56.
[37] PDAC. Briefing document for psychopharmacologic drugs advisory committee (PDAC) meeting of June 9-10, 2009–Quetiapine. Efficacy and safety of Study 149 (D1441C00149). 2009 [June 15, 2012]. URL: http://www.fda.gov/downloads/AdvisoryCommittees/CommitteesMeetingMaterials/Drugs/PsychopharmacologicDrugsAdvisoryCommittee/UCM170736.pdf.
[38] Pandina G, DelBello M, Kushner S, Van Hove I, Augustyns I, Kusumakar V, et al. Risperidone for the treatment of acute mania in bipolar youth [poster]. Boston, MA: Presented at the 54th annual meeting of the American Academy of of Child and Adolescent Psychiatry (AACAP), 2007.
[39] DelBello M, Findling RL, Wang P, Gundapaneni B, Versavel M, eds. Safety and efficacy of ziprasidone in pediatric bipolar disorder. Presented at the Annual Meeting of the American Psychiatric Association; 2008; Washington, DC. May 3-8, 2008.
[40] Delbello MP, Schwiers ML, Rosenberg HL, Strakowski SM. A double-blind, randomized, placebo-controlled study of quetiapine as adjunctive treatment for adolescent mania. J Am Acad Child Adolesc Psychiatry 2002;41(10):1216-23.
[41] Findling RL, McNamara NK, Gracious BL, Youngstrom EA, Stansbrey RJ, Reed MD, et al. Combination lithium and divalproex sodium in pediatric bipolarity. J Am Acad Child Adolesc Psychiatry 2003;42(8):895-901.
[42] Kafantaris V, Coletti DJ, Dicker R, Padula G, Kane JM. Adjunctive antipsychotic treatment of adolescents with bipolar psychosis. J Am Acad Child Adolesc Psychiatry 2001;40(12):1448-56.
[43] Kafantaris V, Dicker R, Coletti DJ, Kane JM. Adjunctive antipsychotic treatment is necessary for adolescents with psychotic mania. J Child Adolesc Psychopharmacol 2001;11(4):409-13.

[44] Kafantaris V, Coletti DJ, Dicker R, Padula G, Pleak RR, Alvir JM. Lithium treatment of acute mania in adolescents: a placebo-controlled discontinuation study. J Am Acad Child Adolesc Psychiatry 2004;43(8):984-93.

[45] Pavuluri MN, Henry DB, Devineni B, Carbray JA, Naylor MW, Janicak PG. A pharmacotherapy algorithm for stabilization and maintenance of pediatric bipolar disorder. J Am Acad Child Adolesc Psychiatry 2004;43(7):859-67.

[46] Biederman J, Mick E, Spencer TJ, Wilens TE, Faraone SV. Therapeutic dilemmas in the pharmacotherapy of bipolar depression in the young. J Child Adolesc Psychopharmacol 2000;10(3):185-92.

[47] Carlson GA, Kelly KL. Manic symptoms in psychiatrically hospitalized children--what do they mean? J Affect Disord 1998;51(2):123-35.

[48] Carlson GA, Bromet EJ, Sievers S. Phenomenology and outcome of subjects with early- and adult-onset psychotic mania. Am J Psychiatry 2000;157(2):213-9.

[49] Scheffer RE, Kowatch RA, Carmody T, Rush AJ. Randomized, placebo-controlled trial of mixed amphetamine salts for symptoms of comorbid ADHD in pediatric bipolar disorder after mood stabilization with divalproex sodium. Am J Psychiatry 2005;162(1):58-64.

[50] DelBello MP, Soutullo CA, Hendricks W, Niemeier RT, McElroy SL, Strakowski SM. Prior stimulant treatment in adolescents with bipolar disorder: association with age at onset. Bipolar Disord 2001;3(2):53-7.

[51] Mota-Castillo M, Torruella A, Engels B, Perez J, Dedrick C, Gluckman M. Valproate in very young children: an open case series with a brief follow-up. J Affect Disord 2001;67(1-3):193-7.

[52] Soutullo CA, DelBello MP, Ochsner JE, McElroy SL, Taylor SA, Strakowski SM, et al. Severity of bipolarity in hospitalized manic adolescents with history of stimulant or antidepressant treatment. J Affect Disord 2002;70(3):323-7.

[53] Pavuluri MN, Janicak PG. Handbook of psychopharmacotherapy: Life span approach. Philadelphia, PA: Williams Wilkins, 2004.

[54] Bowden CL. Lamotrigine in the treatment of bipolar disorder. Expert Opin Pharmacotherapy 2002;3(10):1513-19.

[55] Calabrese JR, Suppes T, Bowden CL, Sachs GS, Swann AC, McElroy SL, et al. A double-blind, placebo-controlled, prophylaxis study of lamotrigine in rapid-cycling bipolar disorder. Lamictal 614 Study Group. J Clin Psychiatry 2000;61(11):841-50.

[56] Wilens TE, Biederman J, Forkner P, Ditterline J, Morris M, Moore H, et al. Patterns of comorbidity and dysfunction in clinically referred preschool and school-age children with bipolar disorder. J Child Adolesc Psychopharmacol 2003;13(4):495-505.

[57] Pavuluri MN, Herbener ES, Sweeney JA. Psychotic symptoms in pediatric bipolar disorder. J Affect Disord 2004;80(1):19-28.

[58] Prince JB, Wilens TE, Biederman J, Spencer TJ, Wozniak JR. Clonidine for sleep disturbances associated with attention-deficit hyperactivity disorder: a systematic chart review of 62 cases. J Am Acad Child Adolesc Psychiatry 1996;35(5):599-605.

[59] Pliszka SR, Greenhill LL, Crismon ML, Sedillo A, Carlson C, Conners CK, et al. The Texas children's medication algorithm project: report of the Texas consensus conference panel on medication treatment of childhood attention-deficit/hyperactivity disorder. J Am Acad Child Adolesc Psychiatry 2000;39(7):908-19.

[60] Smits MG, van Stel HF, van der Heijden K, Meijer AM, Coenen AM, Kerkhof GA. Melatonin improves health status and sleep in children with idiopathic chronic sleep-onset insomnia: a randomized placebo-controlled trial. J Am Acad Child Adolesc Psychiatry 2003;42(11):1286-93.

[61] Saletu-Zyhlarz GM, Anderer P, Arnold O, Saletu B. Confirmation of the neurophysiologically predicted therapeutic effects of trazodone on its target symptoms depression, anxiety and insomnia by postmarketing clinical studies with a controlled-release formulation in depressed outpatients. Neuropsychobiology 2003;48(4):194-208.

[62] Balon R. Sleep terror disorder and insomnia treated with trazodone: a case report. Ann Clin Psychiatry 1994;6(3):161-3.

[63] Rush CR, Baker RW, Wright K. Acute behavioral effects and abuse potential of trazodone, zolpidem and triazolam in humans. Psychopharmacology (Berl) 1999;144(3):220-33.

[64] Brown RT, Amler RW, Freeman WS, Perrin JM, Stein MT, Feldman HM, et al. Treatment of attention-deficit/hyperactivity disorder: overview of the evidence. Pediatrics 2005;115(6):e749-57.

[65] Birmaher B, Axelson DA, Monk K, Kalas C, Clark DB, Ehmann M, et al. Fluoxetine for the treatment of childhood anxiety disorders. J Am Acad Child Adolesc Psychiatry 2003;42(4):415-23.

[66] Fluvoxamine for the treatment of anxiety disorders in children and adolescents. The Research Unit on Pediatric Psychopharmacology Anxiety Study Group. N Engl J Med 2001;344(17):1279-85.

[67] Black B, Uhde TW. Treatment of elective mutism with fluoxetine: a double-blind, placebo-controlled study. J Am Acad Child Adolesc Psychiatry 1994;33(7):1000-6.

[68] Newcorn JH, Schulz K, Harrison M, DeBellis MD, Udarbe JK, Halperin JM. Alpha 2 adrenergic agonists. Neurochemistry, efficacy, and clinical guidelines for use in children. Pediatr Clin North Am 1998;45(5):1099-22, viii.

[69] Graae F, Milner J, Rizzotto L, Klein RG. Clonazepam in childhood anxiety disorders. J Am Acad Child Adolesc Psychiatry 1994;33(3):372-6.

[70] Simeon JG, Ferguson HB, Knott V, Roberts N, Gauthier B, Dubois C, et al. Clinical, cognitive, and neurophysiological effects of alprazolam in children and adolescents with overanxious and avoidant disorders. J Am Acad Child Adolesc Psychiatry 1992;31(1):29-33.

[71] Bernstein GA, Garfinkel BD, Borchardt CM. Comparative studies of pharmacotherapy for school refusal. J Am Acad Child Adolesc Psychiatry 1990;29(5):773-81.

[72] James SP, Mendelson WB. The use of trazodone as a hypnotic: a critical review. J Clin Psychiatry 2004;65(6):752-5.

[73] Pavuluri MN, O'Connor MM, Harral EM, Moss M, Sweeney JA. Impact of neurocognitive function on academic difficulties in pediatric bipolar disorder: A clinical translation. Biol Psychiatry 2006;60(9):951-6.

[74] Geller B, Zimerman B, Williams M, Delbello MP, Frazier J, Beringer L. Phenomenology of prepubertal and early adolescent bipolar disorder: examples of elated mood, grandiose behaviors, decreased need for sleep, racing thoughts and hypersexuality. J Child Adolesc Psychopharmacol 2002;12(1):3-9.

[75] Goldstein TR, Miklowitz DJ, Mullen KL. Social skills knowledge and performance among adolescents with bipolar disorder. Bipolar Disord 2006;8(4):350-61.

[76] Geller B, Craney JL, Bolhofner K, Nickelsburg MJ, Williams M, Zimerman B. Two-year prospective follow-up of children with a prepubertal and early adolescent bipolar disorder phenotype. Am J Psychiatry 2002;159(6):927-33.

[77] Geller B, Bolhofner K, Craney JL, Williams M, DelBello MP, Gundersen K. Psychosocial functioning in a prepubertal and early adolescent bipolar disorder phenotype. J Am Acad Child Adolesc Psychiatry 2000;39(12):1543-8.

[78] Keenan-Miller D, Peris T, Axelson D, Kowatch RA, Miklowitz DJ. Family functioning, social impairment, and symptoms among adolescents with bipolar disorder. J Am Acad Child Adolesc Psychiatry 2012;51(10):1085-94.

[79] Schenkel LS, West AE, Harral EM, Patel NB, Pavuluri MN. Parent-child interactions in pediatric bipolar disorder. J Clin Psychol 2008;64(4):422-37.

[80] Kim EY, Miklowitz DJ, Biuckians A, Mullen K. Life stress and the course of early-onset bipolar disorder. J Affect Disord 2007;99(1-3):37-44.

[81] Rucklidge JJ. Psychosocial functioning of adolescents with and without paediatric bipolar disorder. J Affect Disord 2006;91(2):181-88.

[82] West AE, Weinstein SM. A family-based psychosocial treatment model. Isr J Psychiatry Relat Sci 2012;49(2):86-93.

[83] Pavuluri MN, Graczyk PA, Henry DB, Carbray JA, Heidenreich J, Miklowitz DJ. Child- and family-focused cognitive-behavioral therapy for pediatric bipolar disorder: development and preliminary results. J Am Acad Child Adolesc Psychiatry 2004;43(5):528-37.

[84] West AE, Henry DB, Pavuluri MN. Maintenance model of integrated psychosocial treatment in pediatric bipolar disorder: A pilot feasibility study. J Am Acad Child Adolesc Psychiatry 2007;46(2):205-12.

[85] West AE, Weinstein SM, Peters AT, Katz AC, Henry DB, Cruz R, et al. Child and family-focused cognitive-behavioral therapy for pediatric bipolar disorder: A randomized clinical trial. J Am Acad Child Adolesc Psychiatry 2014;53(11):1168-78.

[86] Fristad MA, Goldberg-Arnold JS, Gavazzi SM. Multifamily psychoeducation groups (MFPG) for families of children with bipolar disorder. Bipolar Disord 2002;4(4):254-62.

[87] Fristad MA, Verducci JS, Walters K, Young ME. Impact of multifamily psychoeducational psychotherapy in treating children aged 8 to 12 years with mood disorders. Arch Gen Psychiatry 2009;66(9):1013-21.

[88] Fristad MA. Psychoeducational treatment for school-aged children with bipolar disorder. Dev Psychopathol 2006;18(4):1289-306.

[89] Miklowitz DJ, George EL, Axelson DA, Kim EY, Birmaher B, Schneck C, et al. Family-focused treatment for adolescents with bipolar disorder. J Affect Disord 2004;82:S113-S28.

[90] Miklowitz DJ, Axelson DA, Birmaher B, George EL, Taylor DO, Schneck CD, et al. Family-focused treatment for adolescents with bipolar disorder: results of a 2-year randomized trial. Arch Gen Psychiatry 2008;65(9):1053-61.

[91] Goldstein TR, Axelson DA, Birmaher B, Brent DA. Dialectical behavior therapy for adolescents with bipolar disorder: a 1-year open trial. J Am Acad Child Adolesc Psychiatry 2007;46(7):820-30.

[92] Hlastala SA, Frank E. Adapting interpersonal and social rhythm therapy to the developmental needs of adolescents with bipolar disorder. Dev Psychopathol 2006;18(4):1267-88.

[93] Hlastala SA, Kotler JS, McClellan JM, McCauley EA. Interpersonal and social rhythm therapy for adolescents with bipolar disorder: treatment development and results from an open trial. Depress Anxiety 2010;27(5):457-64.

In: Mental and Holistic Health: Some International Perspectives ISBN: 978-1-63483-589-3
Editors: J. Calles Jr., D. Greydanus and J. Merrick © 2015 Nova Science Publishers, Inc.

Chapter 7

FEAR AND ANXIETY DISORDERS IN CHILDREN AND ADOLESCENTS

Lauren Boydston[*], *MD, William P French, MD and Christopher K Varley, MD*

Division of Child and Adolescent Psychiatry,
Department of Psychiatry and Behavioral Sciences,
University of Washington School of Medicine, Seattle Children's Hospital,
Seattle, Washington, United States

ABSTRACT

Anxiety disorders are common in children and adolescents and can be quite distressing and impairing for the youth and the family. While some problems with anxiety will resolve on their own, for some youth anxiety can lead to significant impairment in childhood and beyond. Fortunately, effective treatments are available, including cognitive behavior therapy (CBT) and medications such as the selective serotonin reuptake inhibitors (SSRIs). This review will describe common pediatric anxiety disorders and techniques for evaluation and treatment.

INTRODUCTION

Fear and anxiety are normal, and often adaptive, emotional responses to a real or perceived threat. Various worries are typical for children at certain developmental periods (1-3). For example, infants in their first year of life will begin to express anxiety over separation from their primary caregivers, young children often fear the dark and "monsters," and adolescents commonly express high levels of concern about how they are perceived by their peers. For many youth, however, the physical, cognitive and behavioral manifestations of these worries

---

[*] Correspondence: Lauren Boydston, Department of Child Psychiatry, OA.5.154, Seattle Children's Hospital, 4800 Sand Point Way NE, Seattle, WA 98105, United States. E-mail: lauren.boydston@seattlechildrens.org

become excessive in terms of intensity or persistence beyond the typical developmental stage (1-3). When these symptoms become overly distressing and/or impairing to the child, evaluation for an anxiety disorder is indicated. Often, the youth is not able to recognize that his or her worries are excessive or unreasonable, and may therefore present to a primary care provider with a chief complaint of behavioral problems, physical concerns or academic problems, rather than anxiety (1-3).

DEFINITIONS

An overview of the clinical features of anxiety disorders seen in children and adolescents is presented below. Specific criteria for diagnoses are described in detail in the "Diagnostic and statistical manual, 5th edition (DSM-5)" (4). All anxiety disorder diagnoses require the symptoms to be "clinically significant" in terms of the amount of distress or impairment experienced. It is important to note that anxiety disorders are often co-morbid with one another and that, as the child ages, evolving symptom presentations may lead to changes in the specific anxiety diagnosis (1, 2).

Separation anxiety disorder (SAD). Some degree of separation anxiety is normal in infants, and increases in symptoms of separation anxiety may occur transiently with certain events such as starting preschool or kindergarten (1). For children with SAD, the fear of separating from attachment figures is developmentally inappropriate or excessive for the child's age, and must be present for at least 4 weeks (4). A child may avoid age-appropriate activities such as school and sleep-overs. Youth with SAD are likely to express significant distress when they anticipate a separation from home or caregivers. They may worry about events happening that could lead to separation (such as getting lost or kidnapped) or fear that something bad might happen to the caregiver when they are not together (4). As a result, children and adolescents with SAD may be reluctant - or simply refuse - to go anywhere without major attachment figures present. Some children may not want to leave home at all. School refusal is common (2). Nightmares about separation and physical complaints such as headaches and upset stomach may also occur. Caregivers of youth with SAD may experience significant distress as well due to behaviors such as a child's refusal to fall asleep without the parent present, resistance to be cared for by a babysitter, or excessive "clinginess" (4).

Selective mutism. A child with selective mutism refuses to talk in certain situations (4). For example, a child may remain silent throughout the school day but talk normally at home; or, a child may speak to peers and caregivers, but not to other adults. The behavior must go on for at least a month and not be better accounted for by a communication disorder or other disorder in which communication is a significant problem, such as autism (4). A child with selective mutism may be able to use non-verbal communication or written communication to get his or her needs met. Comorbid social anxiety is common (1, 4).

Specific phobia. Specific phobias involve anxiety limited to a particular object or situation, lasting 6 months or more (4). Examples of "phobic stimuli" include spiders, dogs, storms, needles, airplanes, enclosed spaces and heights. Exposure to the trigger causes intense distress, or the youth manages to avoid it altogether (4). Some phobias develop after a specific triggering event, for example intense fear and avoidance of solid food after the child experiences a choking episode. Children may express their fear in an "externalizing manner," for example, by crying or having a tantrum, or they may freeze or cling to a caregiver (4). Fears that are culturally or developmentally normative, or that are realistic for the situation (e.g., going outside at night in a dangerous neighborhood), would not be considered phobias. Before diagnosing a specific phobia, it is important to consider whether the symptoms in question are actually part of another mental disorder such as agoraphobia, obsessive compulsive disorder, social anxiety disorder, an eating disorder, or post traumatic stress disorder (4).

Social anxiety disorder (social phobia). Known by both terms, the core feature is anxiety about social situations. The youth fears being scrutinized, and may think that he or she will do something embarrassing, inadvertently offend someone, be rejected or judged, or act in a way that reveals his or her anxiety (4). The youth experiences intense distress during social situations and may do his or her best to avoid them whenever possible (4). As with other anxiety disorders, the response observed by others may be disruptive behavior, or the youth may "freeze" (4). Examples of feared situations can vary from what may seem to be relatively benign social interactions - such as ordering a drink at a coffee bar or initiating a conversation with a classmate – to more intensive performance situations. To make the diagnosis, the symptoms must be present for at least 6 months (4). The presence of significant distress and impact on social or academic functioning help distinguish social anxiety disorder from shyness, which is not considered pathological (1, 4). A distinction of "performance only type" is made if the anxiety only occurs when the individual is speaking or performing in public (4).

Panic attacks, panic disorder, and agoraphobia. A panic attack involves a sudden sense of fear and/or physical discomfort that reaches peak intensity within minutes. To diagnose a panic attack, 4 of 13 specific symptoms must occur, some of which may be physical (e.g., palpitations, sweating, feeling short of breath) and some of which may be cognitive (e.g., feeling as though things are unreal or that one has become detached from oneself) (4). A panic attack can occur during a time of high anxiety or during a calm state and can be "expected" (that is, there is a clear trigger) or "unexpected" (4). Thus, some panic attacks may seem to come completely "out of the blue," and some sufferers can wake from sleep in a state of panic (1, 2, 4). To meet criteria for panic disorder, at least one of the following conditions must be present: (a) there must be ongoing concern that panic attacks will recur or that they signal something "bad," such as a heart attack; or, (b) the panic attacks have led to a change in behavior, such as avoidance of certain situations due to fears that they could trigger another attack (4). Frequency of panic attacks can vary widely. A youth can experience panic attacks without meeting criteria for panic disorder, and the DSM-5 allows for a panic attack specifier to be attached to any mental disorder (e.g., generalized anxiety disorder with panic attacks, or major depressive disorder with panic attacks) (4).

In the "Diagnostic and statistical manual, 4th edition (DSM-IV)" (5), agoraphobia was only able to be diagnosed when it occurred in the presence of panic disorder. The DSM 5 (4), however, allows agoraphobia to be listed as a separate anxiety disorder diagnosis. Youth with agoraphobia must have significant anxiety related to at least two situations such as use of public transportation, being in open or enclosed spaces, being in a line or crowd, or simply being outside of the home (4). It may be that the youth is worried he or she cannot escape or that he or she will have a panic attack (4). As with separation anxiety, the youth may resist going to school or leaving the home at all; the two diagnoses can be distinguished by the feared outcome (e.g., harm coming to a caregiver in the case of SAD versus embarrassing physical symptoms in the case of agoraphobia) (4).

Generalized anxiety disorder (GAD). The hallmark of GAD is the presence of excessive anxiety and worry that is difficult to control, occurring more days than not, and lasting for at least 6 months (4). In addition, a child experiences at least one additional symptom such as restlessness, fatigue, difficulty concentrating, irritability, muscle tension, and/or sleep problems (4). As with other anxiety disorders, it is not uncommon for youth with GAD to complain of other somatic symptoms, such as frequent headaches or stomachaches (2-4). Unlike other anxiety disorders in which the focus of the worry is often quite consistent, with GAD the youth is likely to have a variety of worries, and the predominant concern may shift from one thing to the next (e.g., grades, having done something wrong, their own or others' health) (1-4). Children with GAD may frequently seek reassurance, constantly redo tasks, and can develop patterns of avoidance and withdrawal from age-appropriate activities (1-4).

Other diagnoses involving anxiety. The diagnosis *unspecified anxiety disorder* can be given to children and adolescents for whom it is not yet clear which specific anxiety disorder best applies (4). For children and adolescents who struggle with significantly impairing and/or distressing levels of anxiety, but who do not meet criteria for one of the specific anxiety disorders listed above, a diagnosis of *other specified anxiety disorder* can be given with an explanation of why the youth does not meet criteria for a more specific diagnosis (e.g., "selective mutism occurring for less than a month" or "recurrent panic attacks limited to only 3 symptoms") (4). When the anxiety is a direct result of a substance or medical disorder, the diagnosis "substance/medication-induced anxiety disorder" or "anxiety disorder due to another medical condition" is given (4).

Anxiety is also a key feature of several disorders that are not classified in the "anxiety disorders" chapter of the DSM-5 (4). These disorders are considered separately because of differences in etiology, core features, course, and/or appropriate treatment. Adjustment disorder with anxiety, acute stress disorder, and post-traumatic stress disorder (PTSD) can all result in significant anxiety symptoms; however, in these cases the development of symptoms is directly related to a specific traumatic or stressful event (4). Youth with obsessive compulsive disorder (OCD) and related disorders, such as trichotillomania, may also experience significant worry and anxiety, and there is significant overlap between the above-described childhood anxiety disorders and OCD-related disorder in terms of treatment (4).

EPIDEMIOLOGY

The prevalence of pediatric anxiety disorders has been estimated to be between 4% and 20% (1-2, 6-8), and it is thought that most adult anxiety disorders have their onset in childhood. In the National Comorbidity Study-Adolescent Supplement (NCS-A) of over 10,000 youth aged 13-18, anxiety disorders were the most common mental health disorders endorsed (9). Thirty-two percent (32%) of adolescents reported having met criteria for at least one anxiety disorder in his or her lifetime, and 8% reported having experienced "severe impairment" from anxiety symptoms. Specifically, 19% of youth endorsed having had a specific phobia, 9% social phobia, 8% SAD, 5% PTSD, 2% panic disorder, 2% GAD, and 2% agoraphobia. In the NCS-

A, half of the youth had developed their anxiety disorder by age 6, with prevalence rates leveling off at about the age of 12. Unfortunately, less than one-in-five of these youth had received any mental health services for his or her anxiety (10).

The prevalence of some disorders, such as SAD, decreases in frequency over time (4). Panic disorder, on the other hand, is rare in children and gradually increases in frequency during adolescence (1). Whereas rates of anxiety disorders are similar in younger boys and girls, they become more common in females by adolescence and into adulthood (11).

Genetics and environmental factors both appear to play important roles in the development of pediatric anxiety disorders. Having a biological relative, particularly a parent, with significant anxiety increases the child's risk (1-2, 4). A temperament characterized by behavioral inhibition - a tendency to avoid things that are new- may predispose a child to development of an anxiety disorder later in life (1-4). Symptoms of an anxiety disorder may start out subclinical with the child tending to worry more or seem more cautious than other children, but without significant distress or functional impairment. Furthermore, anxious caregivers may model anxious coping and unintentionally reinforce behaviors that maintain anxiety, such as avoidance of fear-inducing situations (1). Some anxiety disorders develop following stressful events such as a loss of a loved one or parental divorce (4).

For some children, their anxiety disorder will remit completely (1, 2, 11). For others, the severity of anxiety can wax and wane over time, and the focus of the anxiety may shift as the youth transitions from child to adolescent to adult (1, 2, 11). An individual can struggle with different anxiety disorders at difference times in life (1, 2), for example, meeting criteria for SAD in childhood, social phobia in adolescence, and then developing GAD in adulthood. In addition to the development of new anxiety disorders, children with anxiety are also at increased risk of developing depression (1, 2, 11).

CLINICAL FEATURES

Core DSM 5 criteria and associated clinical features of specific anxiety disorders are described above. As previously stated, knowledge of developmentally-appropriate fears and worries is important in the assessment of anxiety. Anxiety disorders are distinguished from normal worries by the severity and functional impairment or by the inappropriateness for developmental stage (3, 4). Comorbidity between anxiety disorders is common; for example, SAD and GAD often co-occur (2, 4, 11). Comorbidities with other classes of psychiatric disorders are common as well. Youth may also experience clinically significant depression, ADHD, and oppositional defiant disorder (ODD) (1, 2). Providers should be aware that while oppositional behaviors may seem to represent a separate clinical problem, they may in fact be a direct result of the anxiety itself (4). A child may appear non-compliant as he or she attempts to avoid anxiety-inducing situations and may become behaviorally dysregulated as a result of autonomic arousal. Adolescents with anxiety are also at risk of the development of a substance use disorder, including alcohol abuse (1, 2, 11). Although rare in children and adolescents, youth with anxiety should be screened for signs and symptoms of a bipolar spectrum disorder, particularly when medications are being considered.

DIAGNOSIS

The "American Academy of Child and Adolescent Psychiatry" recommends routinely screening for anxiety in any initial mental health assessment (1). Indeed, knowing that anxiety is the most common psychiatric disorder in youth, and knowing that anxiety can present with externalizing behaviors, such as tantrums, it is prudent to consider anxiety any time there is a psychiatric or behavioral chief complaint.

Information should be gathered from both the child and collateral informants (1, 2). Youth typically have the best sense of what is going on internally (1). Adolescents are likely to be able to describe the nature, severity, intensity of their anxiety and associated thoughts and feelings with direct questioning. For young children who have difficulty expressing their internal experiences, strategies such as use of play or drawings, and/or a "feelings thermometer" may be helpful (1, 3). Caregivers and teachers, on the other hand, may be more likely than the child to accurately report any behavioral problems and to describe the functional impact of the anxiety on the child's life (1). Given that comorbidity is common, providers should also screen for symptoms of other common pediatric mental health problems including depression, attentional problems, and disruptive behavior. Providers should ask about the use of prescription and over the counter medications, supplements, caffeinated and other energy drinks, and other substances. Questions should also be asked regarding possible precipitating factors, including traumatic events and peer-related problems such as bullying.

Self- and parent-report rating scales can be very helpful in supplementing the clinical interview, as they allow providers to compare a youth's symptoms to those of a broader population (1). Additionally, some individuals may report symptoms on a checklist that they forgot or did not feel comfortable reporting during the interview. There are multiple "broadband" rating scales available that can be used to screen for multiple types of mental health issues. The "Child behavior checklist" (CBCL), for example, is a well-known and commonly used broadband rating scale that assesses symptoms in multiple domains; it has parent, youth and teacher versions that can be used together to get a more thorough sense of the child's symptomatology and impairment (12). The "Pediatric symptoms checklist-17" (PSC-17) screens for the general categories of "internalizing," "attention" and "externalizing" symptoms (13). In addition to a broadband rating scale, the use of an anxiety-specific rating scale is recommended. The "Screen for child anxiety related emotional disorders" (SCARED), for example, divides anxiety symptoms into various categories that can help delineate specific DSM diagnoses (e.g., panic symptoms or separation symptoms) (14). The SCARED is available in both child and parent versions.

A complete review of systems is recommended to screen for possible medical problems that could be contributing to the anxiety and to document the child's baseline somatic symptoms (1). Because anxiety symptoms can be caused by medical conditions and substances, it is also recommended that the child have a thorough physical examination (11). Laboratory tests such as urine drug screen, thyroid studies, and electrolytes should be considered. Other studies may also be considered based on the nature of the child's physical complaints, e.g., an EKG or Holter monitor for cardiac complaints, a sleep study for ongoing sleep disturbance, or an EEG for symptoms concerning for seizures (2, 11). It is important to note, however, that children with anxiety disorders may be more prone to somatic complaints and have greater difficulty being reassured, which could contribute to a cycle of unnecessary tests and procedures in an attempt to find a "cause." Good clinical judgment, therefore, is essential.

Other medical and psychiatric causes of symptoms should be considered. Medical conditions that can cause anxiety, or mimic some of the features of various anxiety disorders, include hyperthyroidism, hyperparathyroidism, and other endocrine disorders; seizures, central nervous system lesions, migraines and other neurologic conditions; lead poisoning; and asthma (1, 4, 11). Potential substances that can contribute to symptoms of anxiety include medications such as steroids, antiasthmatic medication, antipsychotics, antidepressants, antihistamines, and psychostimulants; drugs of abuse such as methamphetamine, cocaine and even marijuana; caffeine and energy drinks; and withdrawal from agents such as alcohol or benzodiazepines (1, 4, 11). Again, decisions about potential medical investigations should be made in a thoughtful manner to avoid unnecessary and potential harmful interventions.

Other psychiatric conditions have symptoms that overlap with those of the anxiety disorders but should be considered separately, as they may require a much different course of treatment. As noted above, anxious children can appear to have externalizing disorders (e.g., tantrums or disobedience) in their attempt to avoid anxiety-provoking situations; however, for some children these types of behaviors may be unrelated to anxiety and constitute a separate disorder. Core symptoms of autism spectrum disorders, such as the insistence of sameness and ritualized patterns of behavior, can also be confused with anxiety (1, 4). Additionally, the social impairments of youth with higher-functioning autism can be difficult to distinguish from social anxiety; and because the distinction can be subtle, evaluation by a specialist may be necessary. In adolescents, early onset psychosis is a rare cause of anxiety-like symptoms (1, 4). Substance abuse, however, is much more common and should be considered (1, 4, 11).

TREATMENT

Research has shown that there are effective and generally well-tolerated treatments for childhood anxiety disorders, most notably cognitive behavior therapy (CBT) and selective serotonin reuptake inhibitors (SSRIs) (1-3, 6, 11). Some youth will respond well to basic interventions; however, for many, treatment will need to be multimodal and involve coordination between youth, parents, school, primary care providers, and mental health specialists (1).

Education about the nature of anxiety should always be a part of treatment and may need to be ongoing (3). Understanding that anxiety is a normal, adaptive process; learning about the physiological cause of fear and anxiety symptoms; and review of the causes and maintaining factors of anxiety disorders (both in general and for the particular child in question) are important first steps in learning to manage anxiety. How much information to provide the child will of course depend on his or her developmental level.

Psychotherapy. In cases of anxiety that are mild, yet causing some degree of impairment or distress, a psychotherapy-only approach is typically recommended (1). Multiple randomized controlled trials support the efficacy of CBT for anxiety (1, 2, 6, 11). The cognitive (thinking) component of CBT involves teaching children skills to see the association between their thoughts, emotions and behaviors and to challenge their anxious and negative thoughts (1-3, 6). The behavioral component of CBT involves teaching the child and/or parents relaxation skills, imagery, and breathing exercises, and the use of exposure (1-3, 6). Exposure may include the building of a "fear hierarchy," which is used to gradually confront anxiety-provoking stimuli without being allowed to engage in escape behaviors. The positive reinforcement of progress helps increase the likelihood of success (1). For young children, or children with developmental disabilities, treatment will likely entail utilizing more behavioral than cognitive techniques (6). The younger the child, the more heavily parents will need to be involved in the therapy as they will need to help their child practice new skills between sessions and model good anxiety-management skills themselves. There are several CBT manuals for use with youth and adolescents, and for older and/or more cognitively advanced adolescents, manuals meant for adults may also be appropriate. Some adolescents and parents may be able to use self-guided CBT manuals and techniques with good results (1).

Psychodynamic psychotherapy has also been used for decades for the treatment of pediatric anxiety, although there are very few clinical trials testing its efficacy (1). Similarly, there is little empirical evidence for family therapy as a primary treatment for pediatric anxiety disorders (1). In family therapy, the family's structure and/or patterns of interaction are the "patient," rather than one identified individual family member. For some families of anxious children with complicated interpersonal dynamics, combining family therapy with individual CBT for one (or more) family member may be indicated (1).

Classroom interventions for anxious youth may include accommodations, such as more time for assignments or tests and additional support from adults. These accommodations can be written into a 504 or Individualized Education Program (IEP) (1). It is important, however, to be mindful of the possibility of inadvertently reinforcing anxiety by allowing the child to avoid anxiety provoking situations. For example, the ability to do school online at home may be very appealing to some youth with severe anxiety but risks further social isolation and entrenchment of their disorder.

Pharmacotherapy. Medication is considered in cases of moderate to severe anxiety, particularly when there has been no or limited response to psychotherapy, when psychotherapy is not available, or when there is a comorbid problem that is likely to be medication-responsive (1). Studies have supported the efficacy, compared to placebo, of several SSRIs including fluoxetine, fluvoxamine, sertraline, and paroxetine (1, 8, 11). Although none of the SSRIs are US Food and Drug Administration (FDA) approved for the use in non-OCD pediatric anxiety disorders, they are generally considered first-line when medications are used, given the empirical evidence in adults and vast clinical experience (1, 3, 11). There are no studies comparing one SSRI to the other, thus factors in choosing which one to use often include physician and family experience with a particular medication, comorbid diagnoses, and side effect profile (1, 3, 11). Other factors to consider include the FDA approval of the use of fluoxetine, sertraline and fluvoxamine for children with OCD, and the FDA warning issued in 2003 against the use of paroxetine in youth with depression (11).

There is also some evidence supporting the "off label" (i.e., not FDA-approved) use of other medications in pediatric anxiety, such as the selective serotonin and norepinephrine reuptake inhibitor (SNRI) venlafaxine (8, 11). Venlafaxine, however, is generally not used as a first or second choice due to a higher side effect profile (11). Studies comparing tricyclic antidepressants, such as clomipramine or imipramine, in non-OCD anxiety have not been uniformly positive, and because of the potential side effects and risk in overdose compared to

SSRIs, they are infrequently used (1, 2, 11). Data have not supported the use of benzodiazepines in pediatric anxiety, and they carry the possibility of sedation, tolerance, dependence, and adverse effects on learning and memory (1, 11). Thus, they are recommended only for short-term use in severe cases (1, 3, 11), and ideally, on a scheduled rather than as needed basis.

Kodish, and colleagues, proposed an algorithm for medication management of pediatric anxiety based on a review of the available evidence (11). They suggested starting with an SSRI and titrating the dose every 2-4 weeks until there was good response, intolerable side effects, or maximum dose had been reached. If not successful, the next recommended step is to try a second SSRI, followed by venlafaxine. Next, providers could consider buspirone or mirtazapine, either as monotherapy or as augmentation of an SSRI. The use of benzodiazepines was recommended only if necessary for acute symptoms or if all other medication trials were unsuccessful. Table 1 lists the typical starting doses and therapeutic ranges of several medications used for pediatric anxiety.

In a recent study, the SNRI duloxetine was found to be superior to placebo in the treatment of GAD (15). Duloxetine was approved by the FDA for the treatment of GAD in children ages 7-17 in October, 2014 (16). However, clinical experience with duloxetine for pediatric anxiety is still quite limited compared to experience with SSRIs, and it remains to be seen where this medication will fit in standard practice.

Common side effects of SSRIs, such as headaches, nausea and stomachaches, may improve with time (1, 3, 8, 11). These types of symptoms may also occur as a result of the underlying anxiety, so it is important to have a baseline understanding of the child's somatic symptoms. Antidepressants can be activating in some children, so providers should monitor for increased agitation, restlessness, irritability, problems sleeping, worsening anxiety, and/or other behavioral changes (1, 3, 11). Activation from an SSRI should not be confused with a substance-induced manic or hypomanic episode, which is possible with all antidepressants but fortunately very rare (1, 3, 11).

Table 1. Select medications used in the management of pediatric anxiety

Medication	Starting daily dose	Typical therapeutic range
Fluoxetine	5-10 mg	10-60 mg
Sertraline	12.5-25 mg	50-200 mg
Paroxetine	5-10 mg	10-40 mg
Fluvoxamine	12.5-25 mg	100-300 mg divided b.i.d.
Citalopram	5-10 mg	10-40 mg
Escitalopram	2.5-5 mg	5-20 mg
Venlafaxine XR	37.5 mg	75-225 mg
Buspirone	5 mg (b.i.d. or t.i.d)	15-60 mg (divided b.i.d or t.i.d)
Mirtazapine	7.5-15 mg	7.5-30 mg (typically qhs)
Clonazepam	0.25 mg -0.5 mg (q.d.or b.i.d.)	0.25 mg to 3 mg (divided q.d. to t.i.d)
Lorazepam	0.5-1mg	0.5-6 mg (divided q.i.d)

*Not FDA-approved.
Sources 1,3,11.

If considering medications other than SSRIs, be aware of notable side effects such as the potential for venlafaxine to increase blood pressure and for mirtazapine to cause weight gain (11). Since 2004, all medications marketed as antidepressants, including all SSRIs, have been labeled with a "black box warning" about the possible emergence of suicidal thoughts and behaviors (1, 3, 11). This warning emerged from retrospective analysis of studies of youth with depression. In their 2009 review of antidepressant trials for pediatric anxiety, Ipser and colleagues found that only 13 of the 2,519 patients studied experienced suicidal ideation, and there were no completed suicides (8).

When medications are effective, consideration should be given at some point to discontinuation to determine if the medication is still necessary for the child (1). Pine recommends considering a trial off medication after 1 year of improvement, ideally during a low-stress period, such as during summer vacation (17). Given the possibility of withdrawal symptoms and potential increased risk of relapse if stopped abruptly, a gradual taper is recommended (3, 17).

Combination treatment. For children with moderate to severe anxiety, a combination of medication and psychotherapy is recommended (1, 11). If the youth is initially treated with CBT or medication alone without sufficient benefit, then it is recommended that the other component be added to the treatment plan (1, 11). The "Child-adolescent anxiety multimodal study" compared the use of CBT, sertraline, a combination of CBT and sertraline, and a placebo pill in almost 500 youth ages 7 to 17 with SAD, GAD or social phobia (7). After 12 weeks, they found that 80% of youth who received combination treatment were "much or very much improved," compared with 60% who received CBT without medication, 55% who received medication without CBT, and 24% who received placebo.

CONCLUSION

Anxiety disorders are common in children and adolescents. While some problems with anxiety are developmentally appropriate or mild and will resolve on their own, for some youth anxiety can lead to significant impairment in childhood and may portend a life-long struggle - not only with anxiety but with other mental health problems as well. For this reason, it is important to screen for anxiety disorders whenever a child presents with a behavioral or mental-health related complaint, or when anxiety is suspected to be contributing to a physical complaint, and begin treatment when appropriate. There is excellent evidence to support the use of CBT in pediatric anxiety disorders. When CBT is not adequate or when impairment is severe, the combination of medication and therapy may be indicated.

Although use is off-label in non-OCD anxiety, there is a solid base of clinical experience and empirical support for the safe and effective use of SSRIs. Because the response is often robust, treatment of pediatric anxiety disorders can be quite satisfying for the child, family and providers. Additionally, the child and family may develop strategies for anxiety management that benefit them for years to come.

REFERENCES

[1] Connolly SD, Bernstein GA, Work Group on Quality Issues. Practice parameter for the assessment and treatment of children and adolescents with anxiety disorders. J Am Acad Child Adolesc Psychiatry 2007;46:267-83.

[2] Krain AL, Ghaffari M, Freeman J, Garcia A, Leonard H, Pine DS. Anxiety disorders. In: Martin A, Volkmar FR, eds. Lewis's child and adolescent psychiatry: A comprehensive textbook, 4th ed. Philadephia, PA: Wolters Kluwer Health, Lippincott Williams Wilkins, 2007:538-48.

[3] Varley CK, Henry A. Anxiety disorders. In: Greydanus DE, Patel DR, Pratt HD, Calles Jr JL, eds. Behavioral pediatrics, 3rd ed. New York: Nova Science, 2009:239-53.

[4] American Psychiatric Association. Diagnostic and statistical manual of mental disorders, fifth edition. Arlington, VA: American Psychiatric Association, 2013.

[5] American Psychiatric Association. Diagnostic and statistical manual of mental disorders, fourth edition, text revision. Washington, DC: American Psychiatric Association, 2000.

[6] James AC, James G, Cowdrey FA, Soler A, Choke A. Cognitive behavioural therapy for anxiety disorders in children and adolescents. Cochrane Database Syst Rev 2013;6:CD004690.

[7] Walkup JT, Albano AM, Piacentini J, Birmaher B, Compton SN, Sherrill JT, et al. Cognitive behavioral therapy, sertraline, or a combination in childhood anxiety. N Engl J Med 2008;359:2753-66.

[8] Ipser JC, Stein DJ, Hawkridge S, Hoppe L. Pharmacotherapy for anxiety disorders in children and adolescents. Cochrane Database Syst Rev 2009;3:CD005170.

[9] Merikangas KR, He JP, Burstein M, Swanson SA, Avenevoli S, Cui L, et al. Lifetime prevalence of mental disorders in US adolescents: Results from the National Comorbidity Survey Replication—Adolescent Supplement (NCS-A). J Am Acad Child Adolesc Psychiatry 2010;49:980-9.

[10] Merikangas KR, He JP, Burstein M, Swendsen J, Avenevoli S, Case B, et al. Service utilization for lifetime mental disorders in US adolescents: results of the National Comorbidity Survey- Adolescent Supplement (NCS-A). J Am Acad Child Adolesc Psychiatry 2011;50:32-45.

[11] Kodish I, Rockhill C, Ryan S, Varley C. Pharmacotherapy for anxiety disorders in children and adolescents. Pediatr Clin North Am 2011;58:55-72.

[12] Achenbach TM, Ruffle TM. The child behavior checklist and related forms for assessing behavioral/emotional problems and competencies. Pediatr Rev 2000;21:265-71.

[13] Jellinek MS, Murphy JM, Little M, Pagano ME, Comer DM, Kelleher KJ. Use of the Pediatric Symptom Checklist to screen for psychosocial problems in pediatric primary care: a national feasibility study. Arch Pediatr Adolesc Med 1999;153:254-60.

[14] Birmaher B, Brent DA, Chiappetta L, Bridge J, Monga S, Baugher M. Psychometric properties of the screen for child anxiety related emotional disorders (SCARED): A replication study. J Am Acad Child Adolesc Psychiatry 1999;38:1230-6.

[15] Strawn JR, Prakash A, Zhang Q, Pangallo BA, Stroud CE, Cai N, Findling RL. A randomized, placebo-controlled study of duloxetine for the treatment of children and adolescents with generalized anxiety disorder. J Am Acad Child Adolesc Psychiatry 2015;54:283-93.

[16] Mathis MV. Supplemental approval: Fulfillment of postmarketing requirement. Letter. Accessed 2015 May 29. URL: http://www.accessdata.fda.gov/drugsatfda_docs/appletter/2014/021427Orig1s043,s044ltr.pdf.

[17] Pine DS. Treating children and adolescents with selective serotonin reuptake inhibitors: how long is appropriate? J Child Adolesc Psychopharmacol 2002;12:189-203.

Chapter 8

PSYCHIATRIC DISORDERS: OBSESSIVE COMPULSIVE DISORDER

William P French, MD, Lauren Boydston, MD, and Christopher K Varley, MD*

Division of Child and Adolescent Psychiatry,
Department of Psychiatry and Behavioral Sciences,
University of Washington School of Medicine, Seattle Children's Hospital,
Seattle, Washington, United States

ABSTRACT

Obsessive compulsive disorder (OCD) is a psychiatric disorder, which commonly begins in childhood or adolescence, and if inadequately treated, can become chronic and lead to significant functional impairments across the lifespan. Despite the severity of symptoms and impairment, oftentimes it takes years for the disorder to be appropriately identified and treated. Primary care providers (PCPs) can play an important role in identifying OCD through careful history taking and screening. While many PCPs may not feel adequately trained to provide treatment, appropriate referral to specialty providers can lead to favorable clinical outcomes. This review will provide a concise discussion of the typical presentation, assessment, and treatment of OCD in children and will include relevant information regarding its epidemiology, etiology, clinical features, and typical course.

INTRODUCTION

The identification, assessment, and treatment of OCD in primary care settings is challenging on several fronts. First, children and families are often unaware of the core problem behind the symptoms which bring them into their provider's office. For example, rather than

---

[*] Correspondence: William P French, Department of Psychiatry and Behavioral Medicine, M/S OA.5.154, POBox 5371, Seattle Children's Hospital, 4800 Sand Point Way NE, Seattle, WA 98145-5005, United States. E-mail: william.french@seattlechildrens.org

describing a child with intrusive thoughts and compulsive behaviors, parents may present seeking help for explosive tantrums or disruptive behaviors precipitated by an OCD exacerbation. Moreover, the child may intentionally hide his or her symptoms from parents and providers due to embarrassment or shame. Additionally, parents may fail to mention ritualistic behaviors that they assume are developmentally normal, consider them a phase, or they may have gotten so used to the behaviors that they no longer see them as unusual.

A second challenge is that OCD shares comorbidity with a number of other childhood psychiatric disorders, and the majority of patients with OCD have a least one of these. Therefore, unless a child is carefully screened for OCD during the assessment process, signs and symptoms of the illness may be inadvertently attributed to other causes. Lastly, while the best opportunity to identify OCD may be in the primary care setting, optimal treatment will likely require collaboration with specialists who practice in other treatment settings.

Definition

With the 2013 publication of the Diagnostic and Statistical Manual of Mental Disorders, Fifth Edition (DSM-5), OCD is now separately classified from anxiety disorders and is, instead, grouped with several similar disorders, including body dysmorphic disorder and trichotillomania, under the heading OCD and Related Disorders (1). The core definitional components of OCD, however, remain unchanged from the previous edition (DSM-IV TR) and consist of obsessions and/or compulsive behaviors. Obsessions are defined as intrusive, unwanted thoughts, images, or urges that cause distress or worry, which the individual attempts to suppress or ignore through some form of compulsive thought or behavior. Compulsions are defined as repetitive, ritualistic behaviors (e.g., hand washing) or mental acts (e.g., counting), which the individual feels the urge to perform in order to relieve anxiety and distress (1, 2).

A further requirement is that the behaviors are not connected in a realistic way to the worry or problem the individual is trying to prevent or neutralize, or that they are clearly excessive in their intensity or frequency. In older children and adults, the DSM-5 definition requires that the individual have an awareness that the compulsive behaviors are being done with the aim of eliminating unwanted thoughts or urges, but this level of insight is not required for younger children. The definition also stipulates that the unwanted thoughts and compulsive behaviors cause significant functional (e.g., academic) impairment or that they are time consuming (e.g., take more than one hour per day).

Etiology and Epidemiology

The prevalence of pediatric OCD is estimated to be 1% to 2% (3), though estimates of adolescent subclinical OCD range from 4% to 19% (4). Despite OCD commonly being a chronic disease, adult prevalence estimates are less than what would be predicted if the majority of pediatric cases persist through the lifespan, which suggests that a substantial number of childhood-onset cases become subclinical over time (5). Epidemiological studies suggest there are two spikes in the incidence of OCD, one in the early school years, and another in young adulthood (6). If one counts all cases of OCD, the ratio of males to females affected is approximately 1:1; in pediatric OCD, however, males outnumber females 3:2 due to males being more likely to suffer from early-onset OCD (4, 7).

No significant differences in the incidence of OCD have been found among different ethnic or racial groups or geographical regions (4). Pediatric Autoimmune Neuropsychiatric Disorders Associated with Streptococcus (PANDAS), an autoimmune condition thought to cause OCD symptoms through cross reactivity between antibodies to group A B-hemolytic streptococcus (GABHS) and basal ganglia neurons, probably makes up a small subset of all pediatric OCD cases (7).

The etiology of OCD is thought to be multifactorial with various genetic and non-genetic factors likely contributing to the pathogenesis of the disorder (7). Genetic research involving twin studies has shown that concordance rates are higher for monozygotic than dizygotic twins (7). Patients with OCD are more likely than controls to have a first-degree relative with OCD, and interestingly, earlier-onset OCD predicts greater symptom severity in his or her affected first degree relative(s) (8-10). Several putative genetic loci have been identified, and there is evidence that genes regulating the glutamate receptor may have an important role in the etiology of some cases of OCD (11).

Despite this clear evidence that OCD is familial, non-heritable factors are thought to be equally important, which is highlighted by the fact that sporadic OCD cases- those without a clear positive family history- make up the majority of the diagnoses of OCD (7). Nongenetic factors thought to possibly play a role in triggering OCD include in utero exposure to alcohol or tobacco; adverse perinatal experiences, such as maternal infection; and autoimmune responses to infectious agents such as streptococcus (i.e., PANDAS) (12). While PANDAS remains controversial, expert consensus and accumulating evidence is leaning in the direction of validation (7). Furthermore, due to the recognition that other microbes (e.g., mycoplasma) and even non-infectious processes (e.g., metabolic disorders) may play a role in triggering *acute-onset* OCD symptoms, a research group recently proposed modifying the PANDAS criteria and formalizing a broader syndrome called Pediatric Acute-onset Neuropsychiatric Syndrome (PANS) in an effort to capture a wider spectrum of potential etiologic agents implicated in a subgroup of OCD patients with acute-onset symptoms (13).

CLINICAL FEATURES

Pediatric OCD can present in a variety of different ways, which can make proper identification difficult. At times, a trigger or precipitating event may be identified, but it is more likely that symptom onset is insidious (7). Psychiatric comorbidity is estimated at greater than 50% (7), which may result in OCD symptoms being overlooked or associated with the comorbid condition(s). Furthermore, parent accommodation to the symptoms, due a desire to relieve their child's distress (or their own), may have occurred for so long that the parents may underestimate or have a hard time identifying their child's behaviors as being related to OCD (14). Because of this, it may not be the parents, but other adults in the child's life, who first become concerned and push for an evaluation. On average, the time from symptom onset to initial assessment is estimated to be around 3 years (6).

Commonly reported obsessions in youth include contamination concerns, fears of something terrible happening (e.g., death of a parent), need for order or symmetry, and excessive scrupulosity and guilt. Common compulsions include repeated washing, checking, repeating, and ordering (4). While some children present manifesting classic symptoms such as compulsive hand washing due to fear of germs or checking compulsions due to safety concerns, at other times the parents' presenting issues may seem unconnected to OCD (14). For example, parents may complain of extraordinary temper tantrums but not be aware that they typically occur when their child's compulsive rituals are interrupted or prevented (4).

A parent may also have concerns about academic decline and school-related behavioral issues but not realize that perfectionism regarding school assignments, or missed class time due to bathing rituals, is driving the school problems. The fact that children are often either secretive about their symptoms or lack insight or the ability to describe them can contribute to this problem (7). Furthermore, it is important to recognize that while children with OCD often have both obsessions and compulsions, sometimes they present with only one or the other (15).

Thought to be a specific subtype of OCD, PANDAS shares many characteristics of non-PANDAS OCD. Specific clinical features that should cue a clinician to suspect this subtype are preceding or concurrent evidence of streptococcus (or other microbial infection), abrupt (24-48 hours) onset of symptoms, and young age of onset. Sudden-onset tics or other neuropsychiatric symptoms, such as enuresis or emotional lability, although not pathognomonic for PANDAS, are frequently present as well (13).

As stated above, comorbid conditions occur frequently with OCD and may affect clinical presentation, treatment approach, and prognosis. Early-onset OCD increases the risk for attention-deficit/hyperactivity disorder (ADHD), Tourette's disorder, and a wide variety of anxiety disorders (4, 16). Special attention should be given to disorders that can be confused with OCD. Children with autism, for example, are often identified by their parents as obsessive and frequently have repetitive behaviors. However, youth with autism, compared to those with OCD, may seem less concerned or worried about their obsessions and routines (7). Though they often co-occur, OCD also needs to be distinguished from anxiety disorders, such as generalized anxiety disorder (GAD). While both involve excessive worry, compared to OCD, worries in GAD are likely more realistic and generalized to a variety of domains of living (4).

Some youth who eventually develop psychotic disorders initially present with OCD, and these two disorders can appear similar due to the, at times, bizarre nature of particular obsessions and compulsions (7). To help avoid misidentifying individuals with OCD as having a psychotic disorder, DSM-5 includes a specifier, which permits clinicians to identify OCD beliefs as being absent of insight to the extent that they can be considered delusional (1). The fact that the individual demonstrates disordered thinking and impaired reality testing only in the context of his or her specific obsessional concern(s) discriminates delusions in OCD from psychosis (4).

As acknowledged in the DSM-5, there are a number of disorders that appear to be related to, but are distinct from, OCD, such as hoarding, skin picking, hair pulling (trichotillomania), and body dysmorphia. These disorders may occur with, and are sometimes misidentified as, OCD. As in OCD, there is generally a buildup of tension which leads to an urge to perform the behavior but, unlike OCD, there is not clear obsessional content. It is important to consider these disorders separately as they require different treatment approaches (17).

Finally, obsessive compulsive personality disorder (OCPD) shares similarities with OCD but can be distinguished by its stability as a trait (versus the often waxing and waning course of OCD) and by the likelihood that individuals with an OCPD personality style experience their behaviors as ego syntonic (i.e., acceptable and congruent with one's self-image), rather than ego dystonic (i.e., unacceptable and incongruent with one's self-image), as is commonly the case for individuals with OCD (7).

OCD symptom severity commonly waxes and wanes over time, however the original symptom cluster may not be maintained with new symptoms sometimes appearing as others fade (15). The average number of lifetime obsessions and compulsions is 4.0 and 4.8, respectively (15). A National Institute of Mental Health study (18) of 54 patients documented that 43% of subjects still met diagnostic criteria for OCD 2 to 7 years following treatment. While characterized as a chronic, relapsing illness, it is also known that many youth with OCD have symptoms that become subclinical with time or that remit all together. Having specific OCD subtypes (e.g., early onset), comorbid psychiatric illnesses such as ADHD, family dysfunction, and poor insight all predict a poorer response treatment and suggest a worse prognosis.

ASSESSMENT

As previously stated, OCD can be difficult to detect. Therefore, providers should regularly screen for the presence of obsessive thoughts and compulsive behaviors even if a patient's presenting psychiatric or behavioral complaints seem unrelated to OCD. One option for providers is to employ a broadband parent report rating scale such as the Child Behavior Check List (CBCL) (19), which has a number of items shown to have good sensitivity and specificity in identifying OCD symptoms. Screening can also be accomplished by asking several questions related to DSM-5 diagnostic criteria. For example, to screen for obsessive thoughts, a clinician could ask an older child, "Do you ever have unwanted or intrusive thoughts that won't go away that worry you or make you upset?" For younger children, however, the questioning may have to be simplified by asking if they have something that constantly worries them. Additionally, some examples may have to be provided regarding frequently encountered symptoms, such as worries about things being dirty or safety issues (7).

Parents may have to be enlisted to help the child understand what is being asked or to help the child remember times when he or she might have exhibited the behaviors being discussed. When screening for repetitive behaviors or rituals, a clinician may ask about actions a child feels compelled to do over and over to help relieve anxiety even those actions seem strange or do not make sense. When there is a suspicion for the disorder, questions across all major OCD domains should be asked, including contamination fears (e.g., germs), organizing and symmetry (e.g., counting and checking), perfectionism (e.g., redoing homework), hoarding, and excessive scrupulosity and guilt (e.g., confessing and apologizing) (7).

It is important to remember that pre-school, and even school age children, frequently have developmentally normal thoughts and behaviors (e.g., bedtime rituals) that may appear obsessional and compulsive but not be pathological (14). Consideration needs to be given to the frequency, duration, intensity, context, and functional impairment associated with such thoughts and behaviors. To properly screen for the possibility of OCD, questions about previous obsessional thoughts and compulsive behaviors should be asked even if symptoms are not currently present due to the waxing and waning nature of this disorder (14). Clinicians should also ask parents about avoidance behaviors (e.g., refusing to wash a family members' dirty dishes) that may be part of the disease process.

If such screening probes raise the suspicion for OCD, a targeted, comprehensive assessment should be undertaken. There are several formal assessment measures in use, such as the Children's Yale-Brown Obsessive Compulsive Scale (CY-BOCS) (20), which elicits past and present symptoms across major OCD domains and includes a severity scale (21). By asking questions such as time spent in OCD-related behaviors and degree of distress associated with obsessions and compulsions, the severity of illness can rated from mild to severe.

As with any thorough evaluation, a full history needs to be undertaken giving special attention to psychiatry comorbidities and family, medical, and educational history. As previously discussed, comorbidity is the norm rather than exception. Assessment should include screening for common comorbid conditions such as motor and vocal tics. If complex motor tics exist without a history of simple tics, the behavior may be a compulsion. Inquiring as to whether or not there are associated fears or a foreboding of something bad happening if the behavior is not acted upon increases the probability that the behavior is a compulsion rather than a tic (4).

Proper identification of comorbid conditions is not only important from the perspective of adequate treatment but also provides information that can inform the approach to OCD treatment as well. For example, in the Pediatric Obsessive-Compulsive Treatment Study (POTS), when compared to placebo, children with OCD and comorbid tics only benefited from sertraline when it was combined with cognitive behavioral therapy (CBT), whereas children with OCD without tics benefited from sertraline alone (17,22).

While asking about a family history of OCD and common co-occurring illnesses is important, providers should also inquire about current family function and to what degree the illness has led to parental accommodation. Such accommodation is common as parents oftentimes inadvertently reinforce their child's maladaptive behaviors in their effort to relieve his or her anxiety (7). Longstanding high levels of child irritability and maladaptive function can also lead to significant parent-child conflict and overly emotional parental responses in the face of daily struggles.

Medical history should focus on medical conditions associated with OCD symptoms. While PANDAS is the most familiar example, other conditions associated with obsessions and compulsions include carbon monoxide poisoning and Prader-Willi syndrome (4). A recent sore throat or upper respiratory infection, especially in a pre-adolescent with acute-onset symptoms and comorbid tics or other neuropsychiatric symptoms, such as tremor, increases the suspicion for PANDAS (23). If suspected, an adequate throat culture should be obtained along with serial titers for GABHS antistreptoccocal DNAase B and/or antitstreptolysin O antibodies (14). While many non-affected children will be test positive to these antibodies due to previous infections, a doubling of titers over a period of 4-6 weeks indicates an active infection and should be followed by antibiotic treatment (7).

Children with milder forms of OCD may be able to function well in the classroom as long as their specific obsessional and compulsive symptoms do not involve school-related themes.

Academic and behavioral dysfunction at school is often an indication of more severe illness, which may require more immediate and aggressive treatment (7). Neuropsychological testing of children with OCD shows that they often exhibit a specific pattern of impairment, which includes deficits in processing speed, fine motor abilities, and visual capacities (24). In children with OCD and unexplained learning problems, a referral to specialists for appropriate testing may lead to the identification of specific deficits such as these and set the stage for appropriate educational interventions (7).

TREATMENT

A comprehensive, individualized treatment plan is critical to the successful treatment of OCD, as it is enables the primary care provider to match unique individual, family, and illness variables with the most appropriate treatment interventions. Individual factors which may affect treatment include patient age and motivation for treatment (25). Family factors such as overall functional level and degree of accommodation to their child's symptoms are also important to consider. Finally, illness variables such as co-occurring disorders and severity OCD symptoms will also impact treatment planning.

Two types of treatment modalities, cognitive behavioral therapy (CBT) and pharmacotherapy have consistently been shown to be effective in the treatment of OCD (4, 14, 22). While other psychotherapies such as supportive psychotherapy have been applied to the treatment of OCD, only CBT (alone or in combination with medication) has consistently been shown adequate efficacy and acceptability (26, 27). Unfortunately, though numerous treatment manuals and self-help books are available (see ocfoundation.org), qualified therapists may be difficult to locate outside of large urban and academic centers (14). CBT for OCD relies on the traditional elements of CBT but employs an additional component termed "exposure with response prevention (E/RP)," which is considered the most important intervention for successful treatment (4).

Unfortunately, at least according to one clinician survey, up to one third of clinicians who treat pediatric OCD "rarely or never" use E/RP (7). E/RP involves gradually exposing children to situations which increase their anxiety and would typically lead to concomitant compulsive behaviors. Response prevention involves blocking the execution of these behaviors, for example not letting a child wash his or her hands after touching a dirty object. E/RP serves to attenuate anxiety over time, though initially anxiety levels may increase (28). Before children begin E/RP, children and their families receive psychoeducation regarding OCD and treatment principles. Specific symptom targets, realistic goals and barriers to treatment also need to be established (22).

It is extremely important that clinicians build rapport, gain trust, and help children and families understand the importance of learning to be able to tolerate anxiety during this early phase of treatment (14). Without this foundation, later E/RP exposures may be too overwhelming for patients and their families to tolerate, which could lead to noncompliance or withdrawal from treatment. While studies show CBT combined with medications is superior to therapy alone, CBT alone is the preferred treatment for mild to moderate cases of pediatric OCD when possible (7). Predictors of a positive response to CBT alone include low comorbidity, adequate insight, and low levels of family accommodation (7, 29). Conversely, having a first-degree relative with OCD predicts a poor response to CBT alone and favors the combination of CBT and medication, regardless of illness severity (29).

For more severe cases of OCD, best practice guidelines recommend that medication be utilized in combination with CBT (7, 22, 29). The rationale for this recommendation primarily stems from the POTS trial, which showed that CBT combined with sertraline, compared to CBT or sertraline alone, led to a greater reduction in OCD symptoms, as measured on the CY-BOCS. However, a number of factors may justify the use of medications even for milder cases. For example, children with poor insight or motivation, cognitive limitations, or comorbid disruptive behavior disorders may not be good candidates for CBT (7, 25). The lack of readily available quality CBT or severe family dysfunction also may limit non-medication options. Furthermore, when combined with CBT, medications can moderate the increase in anxiety that can be associated with E/RP.

The medications with the best evidence for the treatment of OCD are collectively known as serotonin reuptake inhibitors (SRIs). Clomipramine was the first medication in this class that was given FDA approval for the treatment of OCD in children, and may be clinically superior to the other SRIs in terms of efficacy, but the more favorable risk and safety profiles of the newer selective serotonin reuptake inhibitors (SSRIs) supports their use as first line agents over clomipramine (30-32). SSRIs with FDA approval for the treatment of pediatric OCD include fluoxetine, fluvoxamine, sertraline, and paroxetine. While the SSRIs citalopram and escitalopram do not have FDA approval, they are generally thought to be efficacious as well and may be reasonable choices depending on the clinical situation (14). While clearly superior to placebo with a relatively small number needed to treat of between 4 and 6, less than one half of patients show a clinical response to the first agent tried, and symptom reduction may be modest (7). Response rates are further lowered if there are comorbid illnesses present (17, 22, 29). Therefore, clinicians should make sure patients and parents do not have unrealistic expectations before treatment begins.

Table 1 shows the starting dose and target dose ranges of the SSRIs and clomipramine. Compared to the treatment of depression and anxiety disorders, OCD treatment with SSRIs typically requires higher doses. As is recommended generally with children with depression or anxiety, starting doses should be low and titration rate slow to minimize the likelihood of side effects. While most side effects, if they occur, are mild and transient (e.g., upset stomach, diarrhea, headache), all SSRIs carry a black box warning regarding an increased risk for suicidal ideation and self-harming behaviors, which should be discussed with patients and parents before initiating treatment. Additionally, clinicians should be aware of the possibility of behavioral activation, as well as the potential to cause a medication-induced manic episode in children predisposed to bipolar disorder (33). Serotonin syndrome, though extremely rare, can be life threatening and should be discussed with parents, especially if other serotoninergic agents are being taken.

While titration schedules will vary depending on medication efficacy and tolerability, allowing up to 3 weeks between dose changes allows times for positive medication changes to take place. It may take up to 12 weeks or longer on a SSRI to see if a patient will have an adequate response, so patience is important both for the patient and the provider (7). Also, as stated above, symptom reduction, even with a medication response, may be modest; therefore, clinicians should clearly document baseline symptoms and functioning to track any positive changes that occur over time.

Table 1. SSRIs and clomipramine: typical daily dosing

Medication Name	Starting Dose	Target Doses
Fluoxetine	5-10 mg	10-60 mg
Sertraline	25-50 mg	50-200 mg
Paroxetine	5-10 mg	10-60 mg
Fluvoxamine	25-50 mg	100-300 mg divided b.i.d.
Citalopram	5-10 mg	10-60 mg
Escitalopram	5-10 mg	10-30 mg
Clomipramine	25 mg	100-200 mg

Patients who fail to show a response after an of adequate trial of the maximum recommended dose (or the maximum tolerated) dose of an SSRI, with no change in dose for the preceding 3 weeks, can be considered non-responders and should receive a trial of a second SSRI (7).

Though not a first line agent, clomipramine has utility in patients that are treatment resistant to SSSRIs or as an augmentation agent in partial responders (7). A tricyclic antidepressant with serotonin reuptake blocking properties, clomipramine use requires careful monitoring due to a narrow therapeutic window, potential for significant cardiac side effects, and high lethality in overdose (14, 31). While many of its side effects are relatively mild (e.g., dry mouth, sedation, and dizziness), due to its potential to cause cardiac conduction abnormalities, pre-treatment cardiac examination is recommended, as is baseline and periodic ECG monitoring through the course of treatment with special attention given to QTc prolongation (7, 14). Additionally, it is recommended that serum drugs levels be monitored in order to prevent levels greater than 400 ng/ml (14).

In addition to clomipramine, atypical neuroleptics are sometimes used to augment SSRIs in partial responders or as single agents in children who are treatment resistant. While controlled trials in adults have demonstrated efficacy, none of the atypical agents have FDA approval for OCD or been extensively studied in children with OCD (7). Because of the potential for significant side effects, these agents should be utilized cautiously only after adequate trials of SSRIs have been conducted. Children with comorbid autism spectrum disorder or tics, poor insight, or significant mood instability may the most likely patients to benefit from this augmentation strategy, though weight, glucose, lipids, and the potential for adverse muscle dyskinesias should be closely monitored (34).

The above treatment recommendations regarding CBT and medication interventions apply for OCD symptoms suspected to be PANDAS-related as well. Additional steps, however, need to be taken to adequately treat active streptococcal infections with antibiotics, as stated previously. Relapse, especially if abrupt, should raise concerns for re-infection and prompt a repeat workup and antibiotic treatment if necessary (7, 13, 23). Chronic or severe illness will likely require referral to PANDAS specialists (14).

Children, who adequately respond to medication, either alone or in combination with CBT, should be continued on the medication for at least 12-18 months. If after this period of time, the child remains stable and has only mild symptoms or is symptom free, a slow taper of medication can be entertained (4). If symptoms re-emerge and persist, the medication can be increased to the previous level obtained before the symptoms re-emerged. If the child had previously benefited from CBT, recommending booster sessions may promote a more successful outcome to this process. If after several such trials, the child continues to have relapses, long-term medication treatment may be necessary.

CONCLUSION

Obsessive compulsive disorder (OCD), a psychiatric illness that typically begins in childhood or late adolescence, can be a chronic and debilitating disorder. Though often difficult to detect, proper identification can lead to a favorable outcome as efficacious, evidence-based treatments exist. Treatment usually will not eliminate symptoms but is often effective in reducing morbidity and optimally involves both psychotherapeutic and pharmacological intervention and frequently requires referral to specialty providers.

REFERENCES

[1] American Psychiatric Association. Diagnostic and statistical manual of mental disorders, Fifth Edition. Washington, DC: American Psychiatric Association, 2013.

[2] American Psychiatric Association. Diagnostic and statistical manual of mental disorders, 4th edition, Text Revision (DSMIV-TR). Washington, DC: American Psychiatric Association, 2000.

[3] Flament M, Whitaker A, Rapoport J, Davies M, Berg CZ, Kalikow K, et al. Obsessive compulsive disorder in adolescence: An epidemiological study. J Am Acad Child Adolesc Psychiatry 1988;27:764-71.

[4] Snyder, J. Obsessive compulsive disorder. In: Cheng K, Myers KM, eds. Child and Adolescent Psychiatry: The Essentials. 2nd ed. Philadelphia, PA: Wolters Kluwer Health, Lippincott Williams Wilkins, 2011:140-55.

[5] Stewart SE, Geller DA, Jenike M, Pauls D, Shaw D, Mullin B, et al. Long term outcome of pediatric obsessive compulsive disorder: a meta-analysis and qualitative review of the literature. Acta Psychiatr Scand 2004;110:4-13.

[6] Geller D, Biederman J, Jones J, Park K, Schwartz S, Shapiro S, et al. Is juvenile obsessive compulsive disorder a developmental subtype of the disorder? A review of the pediatric literature. J Am Acad Child Adolesc Psychiatry 1998;37:420-7.

[7] [No authors listed]. Practice parameter for the assessment and treatment of children and adolescents with obsessive-compulsive disorder. J Am Acad Child Adolesc Psychiatry 2012;51(1):98-113.

[8] Do Rosario-Campos MC, Leckman JF, Curi M, Quatrano S, Katsovitch L, Miguel EC, et al. A family study of early-onset obsessive-compulsive disorder. Am J Med Genet B Neuropsychiatr Genet 2005;136B:92-7.

[9] Nestadt G, Samuels J, Riddle M, Bienvenu OJ 3rd, Liang KY, LaBuda M, et al. A family study of obsessive compulsive disorder. Arch Gen Psychiatry 2000;57:358-63.

[10] Pauls D, Alsobrook J II, Goodman W, Rasmussen S, Leckman J. A family study of obsessive-compulsive disorder. Am J Psychiatry 1995;152:76-84.

[11] Hanna GL, Veenstra-Vanderweele J, Cox NJ, Van Etten M, Fischer DJ, Himle JA, et al. Evidence for a susceptibility locus on chromosome 10p15 in early-onset obsessive-compulsive disorder. Biol Psychiatry 2007;62:856-62.

[12] Geller D, Wieland N, Carey K, Vivas F, Petty CR, Johnson J, et al. Perinatal factors affecting expression of obsessive compulsive disorder in children and adolescents. J Child Adolesc Psychopharmacol 2008;18:373-9.

[13] Swedo SE, Leckman JF, Rose NR. From research subgroup to clinical syndrome: modifying the PANDAS criteria to describe PANS (Pediatric Acute-Onset Neuropsychiatric Syndrome). Pediatr Therapeut 2012; 2:113.

[14] Henry A, Varley CK. Obsessive compulsive disorder. In: Greydanus DE, Patel DR, Pratt HD, Calles JL, eds. Behavioral pediatrics. 3rd ed. New York: Nova Science, 2009:255-62.
[15] Rettew DC, Swedo SE, Leonard HL, Lenane MC, Rapoport JL. Obsessions and compulsions across time in 79 children and adolescents with obsessive-compulsive disorder. J Am Acad Child Adolesc Psychiatry 1992;31:1050-6.
[16] Geller D, Biederman J, Faraone SV, Bellorde CA, Kim GS, Hagermoser LM. Disentangling chronological age from age of onset in children and adolescents with obsessive compulsive disorder. Int J Neuropsychopharmacol 2001;4:169-78.
[17] March J, Franklin M, Leonard H, Garcia A, Moore P, Freeman J, et al. Tics moderate treatment outcome with sertraline but not cognitive-behavior therapy in pediatric obsessive-compulsive disorder. Biol Psychiatry 2007;61:344-7.
[18] Leonard HL, Lenane MC, Swedo SE, Rettew DC, Gershon ES, Rapoport JL. Tics and Tourette's disorder: a 2- to 7-year follow-up of 54 obsessive-compulsive children. Am J Psychiatry 1992;149(9):1244-51.
[19] Achenbach TM. Manual for the Child Behavior Checklist 4–18 and 1991 Profile. Burlington, VT: University of Vermont Department of Psychiatry, 1991.
[20] Scahill L, Riddle M, McSwiggin-Hardin M, et al. Children's Yale-Brown Obsessive Compulsive Scale: reliability and validity. J Am Acad Child Adolesc Psychiatry 1997;36:844-852.
[21] Scahill L, Riddle M, McSwiggin-Hardin M, Ort SI, King RA, Goodman WK, et al. Children's Yale-Brown Obsessive Compulsive Scale: reliability and validity. J Am Acad Child Adolesc Psychiatry 1997;36:844-52.
[22] Pediatric OCD Treatment Study (POTS) Team. Cognitive-behavior therapy, sertraline, and their combination for children and adolescents with obsessive-compulsive disorder: the Pediatric OCD Treatment Study (POTS) randomized controlled trial. JAMA 2004;292(16):1969-76.
[23] Swedo SE, Leonard HL, Garvey M, Mittleman B, Allen AJ, Perlmutter S, et al. Pediatric autoimmune neuropsychiatric disorders associated with streptococcal infections: clinical description of the first 50 cases. Am J Psychiatry 1998;155(2):264-71.
[24] Andres S, Boget T, Lazaro L, et al. Neuropsychological performance in children and adolescents with obsessive-compulsive disorder and influence of clinical variables. Biol Psychiatry 2007;61:946-51.
[25] Storch EA, Merlo LJ, Larson MJ, Geffken GR, Lehmkuhl HD, Jacob ML, et al. Impact of comorbidity on cognitive-behavioral therapy response in pediatric obsessive compulsive disorder. J Am Acad Child Adolesc Psychiatry 2008;47:583-92.
[26] March JS, Mulle K. OCD in Children and Adolescents: A Cognitive-Behavioral Treatment Manual. New York: Guilford, 1998.
[27] Watson HJ, Rees CS. Meta-analysis of randomized, controlled treatment trials for pediatric obsessive-compulsive disorder. J Child Psychol Psychiatry 2008;49:489-98.
[28] Foa EB, Kozak MJ. Emotional processing of fear: exposure to corrective information. Psychol Bull 1986;99:20-35.
[29] Garcia AM, Sapyta JJ, Moore PS, Freeman JB, Franklin ME, March JS, et al. Predictors and moderators of treatment outcome in the Pediatric Obsessive Compulsive Treatment Study (POTS I). J Am Acad Child Adolesc Psychiatry 2010;49:1024-33.
[30] Biederman J. Sudden death in children treated with a tricyclic antidepressant: a commentary. J Am Acad Child Adolesc Psychiatry 1991;30:495-7.
[31] Flament MF, Rapoport JL, Berg CJ, Sceery W, Kilts C, Mellström B, et al. Clomipramine treatment of childhood obsessive-compulsive disorder: a double-blind controlled study. Arch Gen Psychiatry 1985;42:977-83.
[32] March JS, Biederman J, Wolkow R, Safferman A, Mardekian J, Cook EH, et al. Sertraline in children and adolescents with obsessive-compulsive disorder: a multicenter randomized control trial. JAMA 1998;280:1752-6.

[33] Martin A, Young C, Leckman JF, Mukonoweshuro C, Rosenheck R, Douglas L. Age effects of antidepressant-induced manic conversion. Arch Pediatr Adolesc Med 2004;158:773-80.

[34] McDougle C, Epperson C, Pelton G, Wasylink S, Price L. A double-blind placebo-controlled study of risperidone addition in serotonin-reuptake inhibitor-refractory obsessive–compulsive disorder. Arch Gen Psychiatry 2000;57:794-801.

SECTION TWO: A HOLISTIC WORLDVIEW

In: Mental and Holistic Health: Some International Perspectives   ISBN: 978-1-63483-589-3
Editors: J. Calles Jr., D. Greydanus and J. Merrick   © 2015 Nova Science Publishers, Inc.

Chapter 9

WORLD HEALTH ORGANIZATION MODEL LIST OF ESSENTIAL MEDICINES

Søren Ventegodt, MD, MMedSci, EU-MSc-CAM[1,2,3,*]

[1]Quality of Life Research Center,
[2]Research Clinic for Holistic Medicine,
[3]Nordic School of Holistic Medicine,
Copenhagen, Denmark

ABSTRACT

The author has reviewed the World Health Organization's (WHO) drug directories and found they are based on data from the pharmaceutical industry's own documentation files and not from studies of higher quality, i.e. meta-analyses from independent researchers such as the Cochrane reviews. Many drugs recommended in WHO's drug directories that are listed as "essential medicines" are found in Cochrane reviews to be without significant positive effects, but causing a number of often severe adverse effects, including sexual problems, heart problems, and even sudden death. As WHO has been acknowledged as a world leader in medicine, its 194 member states are likely to follow WHO's recommendations. The bias found in the WHO drug directories are also found in the national Danish drug directories and we believe that there is a causal relationship here as Denmark follows WHO's recommendations. We also believe that this pattern is present in most if not all of WHO's 194 member states. As WHO's recommendations are passed on to various countries, doctors, and patients by their national health authorities, we estimate that the treatment of people in at least the major cities of the wealthy member states are influenced by the biased information coming from WHO; this group are the patients who can afford to buy these drugs and is estimated at three billion person. We estimate that at least 100,000,000 patients today are treated with pharmaceutical drugs that have no or almost no beneficial effect but often have many harmful adverse effects. We recommend a fundamental revision of WHO and warn all governments, physicians, and patients that the existing WHO drug directories are strongly biased and not reliable sources of information on drugs, vaccines, and other medicines. We encourage all 194

---

[*] Correspondence: Søren Ventegodt, MD, MMedSci, EU-MSc-CAM, Director, Quality of Life Research Center, Frederiksberg Allé 13A, 2tv, DK-1661 Copenhagen V, Denmark. E-mail: ventegodt@livskvalitet.org

WHO member states to use their power as member states to revise this malfunctioning WHO system.

INTRODUCTION

The World Health Organization (WHO) gives recommendations on medicine to its 194 member states. These recommendations come in lists and directories over useful, necessary, and "essential" medicines. We have analyzed WHO's drug directory (WHO's Model List of Essential Medicines) (1) and found that it, like the national Danish drug directory "medicine.dk" we have analyzed earlier (2), is based on information from industrial drug trials instead of on the more objective and reliable information on pharmaceutical drugs provided by meta-analyses made by researchers independent of the pharmaceutical industry, such as the Cochrane reviews from the Cochrane collaboration.

Whole classes of drugs that in independent meta-analyses have been found to be of little clinical value, or even harmful and of no value as medicine; however, they are still listed in the WHO drug directories as beneficial pharmaceutical drugs, including cytotoxic anti-cancer chemotherapy (3-5), the anti-depressive drugs (6), the anti-psychotic drugs (7), the influenza vaccines (8) and the anti-influenza medicines (9). Table 1 compares the NNTs and NNH_{total}s from the two different sources for selected groups of pharmacological drugs.

THE COCHRANE COLLABORATION POSITION

A number of meta-analyses and Cochrane reviews have recently documented that the drugs are less useful than generally assumed. The pharmaceutical drugs used by psychiatry are in general not helping the patients but only harming them according to the Danish leader of the Nordic Cochrane Center, Peter Gøtzsche. In the major Danish daily newspaper, Politiken, he recently concluded that "Our citizens would be far better off if we eliminated all psychopharmacological drugs from the market because doctors are not able to handle them" (10).

In his article Gøtzsche points out that antidepressants cause suicide in patients under 40 years old, causes bipolar disorder in children, gives a majority of the patients sexual problems, and makes people dependent on them. Also noted is that antipsychotic drugs are normally not necessary not even with schizophrenic patients; such drugs prolong the time the patients are sick, create chronic patients, and they are the major reason why schizophrenic patients live 20 years shorter than other people (10). In this way the psychiatric treatment by psychopharmacological drugs has itself become the major cause of health problems, quality of life problems, disease, and even death and suicide for the mentally ill.

That this bad news comes from a leader of a movement with 3000 researchers who are making high quality research independent of the pharmaceutical industry is extremely alarming, and the big media in Denmark and other countries are now debating how to improve the state of medicine. It is worth noticing that Denmark seems to be using the drugs and drug classes recommended by WHO.

Table 1. NNT, NNH$_{total}$ and (Therapeutic Value TV= NNH$_{total}$/NNT) for groups of pharmaceutical drug. Data coming from industrial trials are compared with data from independent meta-analyses. WHO's recommendations in its drug directories are in accordance with the industrial data and in conflict with the data from the independent reviews. All the listed types of pharmaceutical drugs are recommended by the WHO (1)

Drug-class (with outcome)	Typical numbers from industrial trials seemingly used by WHO as basis for recommendations in drug directories (see text)			Typical numbers from Cochrane/reviews seemingly not used by WHO and conflicting with WHOs recommendations in WHO's drug directories (see text)			(ref)
	NNT ;	NNH$_{total}$*) ;	TV**	NNT ;	NNH$_{total}$;	TV	
Antidepressant drugs (outcome: less depressed)	3-20;	2-4;	≈1	∞;	1;	0	((6), Note 1)
Antipsychotic drugs (outcome: mental state improved)	3-20;	2-4;	≈1	∞;	1;	0	((7), Note 2)
Cytotoxic anticancer chemotherapy (outcome: better survival, treatment vs. no treatment)	10-100 ;	1 ;	0.1-0.01	∞;	1;	0	((3-5), Note 3)
Cytotoxic anticancer chemotherapy (outcome quality of life improved, treatment vs. no treatment)	10-100 ;	1 ;	0.1-0.01	∞;	1;	0	((3-5), Note 4)
Anti-influenza medicine (outcome: Influenza prevented)	10-50 ;	1-5 ;	≤0.5	∞;	1;	0	((9), Note 5)
Influenza vaccines (outcome: Influenza prevented)	10-50 ;	1-5 ;	≤0.5	∞;	1-3;	0	((8), Note 6)

*) The size of NNHtotal is often determined by a few very common side effects, so NNH is often a third or so of NNH$_{total}$.
**) TV ("Therapeutic value") expressing the balance between beneficial and harmful effects of a drug or medicine is calculated as NNH$_{total}$/NNT (NNH$_{total}$ is the Number of patients Needed to Treat for one patient to have one adverse effect/ NNH$_{total}$/NNT is the Number of patients Needed to Treat for one patient to have a beneficial effect).
Note 1: The effect can be explained as active placebo.
Note 2: The only relevant outcome for the patients is the improvement of "mental state" (or quality of life) but this was found not improved.
Note 3: It was found that chemotherapy shortened the patients' life; since this study has data comparing treatment with no treatment not been collected by the pharmaceutical industry.
Note 4: It was found that chemotherapy destroyed the patients' quality of life; since this study has data comparing treatment with no treatment not been collected by the pharmaceutical industry.
Note 5: Influenza vaccines were found not useful.
Note 6: Anti influenza drugs were found not useful and very harmful.

RANKING OF MEDICAL SCIENCE ACCORDING TO QUALITY

The consequence of WHO still using the industrial data and not the data from studies of higher quality is a strong bias so the pharmaceutical drugs are generally presented as being more beneficial and less harmful than they actually are; this leads to misinformation for the 194 WHO member states and the public.

Even ranking the scientific studies' quality has been an issue of debate; the pharmaceutical industry has defended its use of the RCT method that recently has been strongly criticized by researchers in methodology such as the leaders of the Cochrane collaboration (11-13).

Table 2 gives our recommendation for ranking study quality based on the conclusions from the Cochrane Collaboration's most recent examinations of the RCT method (11-14). Only science of level 1 and 2 supplies valid and unbiased information on medicine; while cohort studies are more reliable, they are often costly and they often take many years while before-and after studies can be done quickly and on a low budget.

Table 2. Evidence Level 1-11 (after study quality) of drug trials. The reliability of the trial varies significantly with the level of analysis (RCT, review of RCTs, meta-analysis of RCTs, national study, cohort study) and the level of independency from the pharmaceutical industry (1 is best and most reliable, 11 worst and least reliable)

1. Cohort studies of long term positive and negative effects of pharmaceutical drugs on the different categories of patients made by independent researchers at independent research centers. Data i.e. design of questionnaires must be collected independently of commercial interest, and important factors like global quality of life, self-assessed physical and mental health, and survival must be included. All types of medicine the patients have used including non-drug medicine must also be included. Academic experts may have often open or hidden ties to the pharmaceutical industry which can give severe bias also to data from cohort studies and central registers.
2. Simple before and after studies of treatment versus no treatment (including at least 20 patients and 20 controls in non-drug studies and at least 2000 patients and 2000 controls in drug studies) where important factors like global quality of life, self-assessed physical and mental health, and survival are included, and all side/adverse effects are listed and controlled for, and done by independent researchers at independent research institutions. Studies of chronic patients can use the patients as their own control.
3. Studies by independent researchers at independent research centers based on data from national studies using central registers made by independent researchers at independent research centers. If the health organizations of the state are influenced by the pharmaceutical industry, which is often the case, the data and also the studies based on them will be biased.
4. Meta-analyses of meta-analyses of RCTs made by independent researchers at independent research centers (studies including several meta-analyses). If the data comes from RCTs made by researchers related to the pharmaceutical industry, they are biased, and all analyses no matter how objective, will still be biased and not reliable. If an active chemical substance is used as medicine the placebo used for control MUST be active placebo; if not the result is not reliable.
5. Reviews of meta-analyses of RCTs made by independent researchers at independent research centers. If the data comes from RCTs made by researchers related to the

pharmaceutical industry, they are biased, and all analyses no matter how objective, will still be biased and not reliable.
6. Meta-analyses made by independent researchers at independent research centers i.e. the Cochrane reviews are as good as the data is. If the data comes from RCTs made by researchers related to the pharmaceutical industry, they are biased, and all analyses no matter how objective, will still be biased and not reliable. This is a problem for most Cochrane reviews.
7. Reviews of RCTs made by independent researchers at independent research centers i.e. the Cochrane reviews are as good as the data is. If the data comes from RCTs made by researchers related to the pharmaceutical industry, they are biased.
8. Cohort studies of long term positive and negative effects of pharmaceutical drugs on the different categories of patients made by physicians, statisticians and other experts paid or in any other ways supported by the pharmaceutical industry are biased; they are made to serve the one who pays and not a reliable source of information.
9. Data from central registers collected by independent experts are good but studies made by physicians, statisticians and other experts paid or in any other ways supported by the pharmaceutical industry or made in institutions supported by or working together with the pharmaceutical industry are biased. Academic experts have most often open or hidden ties to the pharmaceutical industry so data from central registers using their services are biased.
10. Meta-analysis of RCTs made by physicians, statisticians and other experts paid or in any other ways supported by the pharmaceutical industry are biased and not reliable.
11. RCTs are in general not reliable due to methodological problems (6, 11, 12, 13, 14, 33, 34); bias can too easily be introduced through the many phases of the procedure. RTCs sponsored by pharmaceutical companies are therefore always severely biased and not a reliable source of information. RCTs made by organizations or national agencies which members are supported by or related to the pharmaceutical industry are biased. RCTs made by members of academic institutions who are supported by pharmaceutical companies are biased. RCTs approved by a Scientific Ethical committee without sufficient expertise in RCTs and scientific test methods are likely to be biased.

THE CONSEQUENCES OF BIAS IN THE WHO DRUG DIRECTORIES

Denmark seems to be following WHO's recommendations closely; we therefore find it likely that the similar bias in the national Danish drug directory we have documented earlier (2) is directly or indirectly inherited from the bias we now find in the drug directories of WHO. We believe that this problem systematically impacts all the 194 WHO member states.

The consequence of WHO misguiding its 194 member states seems to be that at least 100,000,000 patients are getting the wrong treatment. This number is estimated from the number of patients who 1) live in the major cities of the wealthy member states (about 3 billion people) and 2) who are sick (about 1 billion) and 3) who are treated with one of the ineffective and dangerous pharmaceutical drugs (from the groups in table 1) by their doctors following the flawed WHO recommendations passed on to them by the local health authorities (at least 10% or 100.000.000 patients - in many wealthy countries like Denmark about 35%).

These patients are thus being treated with pharmaceutical drugs *which have a scientifically documented lack of positive effect and a scientifically documented presence of one or more adverse effects.* These drugs are thus only harmful and not beneficial to these patients.

OBJECTIVE INFORMATION

In order to make physicians and patients able to choose the optimal treatment for a clinical condition WHO should provide objective information about medicine. As the concept "medicine" covers both pharmaceutical, surgical, and therapeutic treatments with non-invasive, non-pharmacological medicine (talk and touch therapy) WHO should also include the existing information about evidence-based non-drug medicine (i.e. from (15-20) in its directories.

Table 3. NNT and NNH$_{total}$ numbers for the best evidence-based non-drug treatments of physical and mental disorders, quality of life and sexual-health issues, and working disability (mostly based on clinical studies using chronic patients as their own control i.e. based on studies of level-2 quality, see 15-29 for reviews). Only data on the most important clinical conditions are listed

NON-DRUG MEDICINE for physical health			
Subjectively poor physical health	NNT=1-3	NNH and NNH$_{total}$>10.000 [*]	TV>10.000 (22)
Coronary heart disease	NNT=1-2	NNH and NNH$_{total}$>10.000 [*]	TV>10.000 (32,33)
Cancer (QOL)	NNT=1-3	NNH and NNH$_{total}$>10.000 [*]	TV>10.000 (23,34)
Cancer (survival)	NNT=2-20	NNH and NNH$_{total}$>10.000 [*]	TV>10.000 (23,34)
Chronic pain	NNT=1-3	NNH and NNH$_{total}$>10.000 [*]	TV>10.000 (22,25)
NON-DRUG MEDICINE for mental health			
Mental health problems in general	NNT=1-3	NNH and NNH$_{total}$>10.000 [*]	TV>10.000 (16-18)
Schizophrenia	NNT=2-5	NNH and NNH$_{total}$>10.000 [*]	TV>10.000 (16-18,26)
Major depression	NNT=1-3	NNH and NNH$_{total}$>10.000 [*]	TV>10.000 (16-18)
Anorexia Nervosa	NNT=1-3	NNH and NNH$_{total}$>10.000 [*]	TV>10.000 (16-18)
Anxiety	NNT=1-2	NNH and NNH$_{total}$>10.000 [*]	TV>10.000 (16-18)
Social phobia	NNT=1-3	NNH and NNH$_{total}$>10.000 [*]	TV>10.000 (16-18)
NON-DRUG MEDICINE for sexual dysfunctions			
Subjectively poor sexual functioning (both gender)	NNT=1-2	NNH and NNH$_{total}$>10.000 [*]	TV>10.000 (see 19)
Male erectile dysfunction	NNT=1-2	NNH and NNH$_{total}$>10.000 [*]	TV>10.000 (see 19)
Female orgasmic dysfunction	NNT=1-2	NNH and NNH$_{total}$>10.000 [*]	TV>10.000 (see 19)
Female lack of desire	NNT=1-3	NNH and NNH$_{total}$>10.000 [*]	TV>10.000 (see 19)
Female dyspareunia	NNT=1-3	NNH and NNH$_{total}$>10.000 [*]	TV>10.000 (see 19,29)
Vaginismus	NNT=1-3	NNH and NNH$_{total}$>10.000 [*]	TV>10.000 (see 19,29)
Vulvodynia	NNT=1-2	NNH and NNH$_{total}$>10.000 [*]	TV>10.000 (see 19,29)
Infertility (closed ovarian tubes)	NNT=3	NNH and NNH$_{total}$>10.000 [*]	TV>10.000 (see 19,29)
NON-DRUG MEDICINE for psychological and existential problems			
Subjectively poor quality of life	NNT=1-2	NNH and NNH$_{total}$>10.000 [*]	TV>10.000 (16-18,26)
Low sense of coherence	NNT=1-3	NNH and NNH$_{total}$>10.000 [*]	TV>10.000 (26)
Suicidal prevention (with decisions)	NNT=1	NNH and NNH$_{total}$>10.000 [*]	TV>10.000 (26)
Low self-esteem	NNT=1-2	NNH and NNH$_{total}$>10.000 [*]	TV>10.000 (16-18)
NON-DRUG MEDICINE for low working ability			
Subjectively poor working ability	NNT=2	NNH and NNH$_{total}$>10.000 [*]	TV>10.000 (26)

[*] According to the many Cochrane reviews in (15) are side effects extremely rare in non-invasive non-drug medicine, like talk-therapy and massage, estimated one in a million patients (i.e. short reactive psychosis). High-energy manipulation like Chiropractic are known to have more side effects (i.e. fractures) but they are still rare (NNH$_{total}$ > 1000).

If one compare the NNT and NNH numbers for the drug treatments and non-drug treatments, it is clear that the non-invasive non-drug treatments using only touch and talk therapy are often favourable, especially if the two methods are combined. Such "holistic" treatments with emotionally oriented bodywork (19-21) and psychodynamically oriented psychotherapy (16-18, 22) are in general highly effective and almost without side effects (see table 3, based on studies of level-2 quality (comp. table 2)) (see 15-29 for reviews).

NUMBER NEEDED TO TREAT (NNT) AND NUMBER NEEDED TO HARM (NNH)

Remember that NNT numbers for pharmaceutical drugs are normally 20 or higher (29), meaning that only one patient in 20 (i.e. 5% of the patients!) or even less is helped by these drugs. NNH numbers of drugs are often 2-5 and as a drug often have many adverse effects; the NNH_{total} numbers are often around 1, meaning that in average every patient using the drug will have an adverse effect.

When we compare the drug treatments with non-drug medicine, it seems that such treatments are in general far more effective and far less dangerous than a treatment with drugs (or surgery). If WHO published the NNT, NNH, NNH_{total} and TV numbers for the pharmacological drugs, surgical interventions, and the evidence-based non-drug treatments for every clinical condition for comparison, we believe that very few doctors and patients would chose a drug treatment in the future. In general a non-drug non-invasive treatment must be recommended for most clinical conditions if you base recommendations on the best scientific evidence.

Some of the drugs recommended by WHO (especially the drugs used in psychiatry such the antipsychotic drugs) are not only causing sexual and other quality of life problems but according to leaders of the Cochrane collaboration (11) and also a national Danish report (31), they are documented to cause heart problems (NNH≈20) and even the patient's sudden death (NNH≈1000). Such drugs have according to estimates from leaders of the Cochrane collaboration already caused the death of thousands of patients worldwide (11) but WHO continues to recommend them. Also, patients with cancer and coronary heart disease are often getting a medical treatment which is not the best, safest and most effective according to the newest medical evidence on the efficacy and harm of the psychotherapy, bodywork, psychosomatic treatments, and CAM-interventions (15-35) (comp. table 1 with table 3).

CORE PRINCIPLES

In order to solve the serious problem that WHO's drug directories are biased and that WHO therefore is seriously misleading its member states, millions of doctors, and a billion patients, we have identified the core principles for rational listening of data regarding positive and negative effects of the pharmaceutical drugs and medicines in general (see table 4) (improved from (2). An outline of a standard list of positive and negative drug (or treatment) effects is suggested here.

Information on each drug should be provided with due regard to dose, indication of use, all clinically relevant outcomes, method of drug study used for documentation, including placebo type, and the quality of the study.

Table 4. Structure of table for listing the positive and negative effects and therapeutic value of pharmaceutical drugs, vaccines, surgeries, examinations, and medicines and medical procedures in general.
(When a surgical intervention or a non-invasive non-drug medicine is listed, the name of the treatment/cure and the applied intensity replaces the word "drug" in the list i.e. "Swedish massage, one weekly session"). For practical reasons the medicine directory must have one entrance for the treatment/cure to see what it is good for, and one entrance for the clinical condition, to see what can cure it. Here we only show how to make the first list

Drug A, dose α

    A α 1. Indication: Disease D1

		Short term	Medium term	Long term
Positive effects (Benefit)				
A α 1-B(1)				
Outcome 1: XXX.	NNT	X	X	X
Method of documentation:		a/b/c/d	a/b/c/d	a/b/c/d
Evidence level (1-11)		N	N	N
	Reference	(1,2,3…)	(6,7,8…)	(12,13,14…)
A α 1-B(2)				
Outcome 2: XXX.	NNT	X	X	X
Method of documentation:		a/b/c/d	a/b/c/d	a/b/c/d
Evidence level (1-11)		N	N	N
	Reference	(21,22,23…)	(26,27,28…)	(32,33,34…)
ETC				
Negative effects (Harm)				
A α 1-H(1)				
Adverse effect 1: XXX.	NNH	X	X	X
Method of documentation:		a/b/c/d	a/b/c/d	a/b/c/d
Evidence level (1-11)		N	N	N
	Reference	(41,42,43…)	(46,47,48…)	(52,53,54…)
A α 1-H(2)				
Adverse effect 2: XXX.	NNH	X	X	X
Method of documentation:		a/b/c/d	a/b/c/d	a/b/c/d
Evidence level (1-11)		N	N	N
	Reference	(61,62,63…)	(66,67,68…)	(72,73,74…)

Table 4. (Continued)

A α 1-H(3)							
Adverse effect 3: XXX.	NNH	X	X	X			
Method of documentation:		a/b/c/d	a/b/c/d	a/b/c/d			
Evidence level (1-11)			N	N	N		
			Reference	(81,82,83…)	(86,87,88…)	(92,93,94…)	
ETC							
A α 1-H (Death)							
Death	NNH	X	X	X			
Method of documentation:		a/b/c/d	a/b/c/d	a/b/c/d			
Evidence level (1-11)			N	N	N		
			Reference	(121,122,123…)	(126,127,128…)	(132,133,134…)	
A α 1-H (total)							
Total harm	NNH$_{total}$	X	X	X			
Method of documentation:		a/b/c/d	a/b/c/d	a/b/c/d			
Evidence level (1-11)			N	N	N		
			Reference	(221,222,223…)	(226,227,228…)	(232,233,234…)	

Therapeutic value (Benefit/Harm)

Estimated therapeutic value for the treatment of disease 1 with drug A, dose α:

	Short term	Medium term	Long term
Therapeutic value (NNT/NNH$_{total}$)	X	X	X

A α 2. Indication: Disease D2

                                Short term Medium term Long term

      ETC

A α 3. Indication: Disease D3

                                    Short term Medium term Long term

      ETC

Drug A, dose β

ETC

Drug A, dose μ

ETC

Drug B, dose α

ETC

…

REFERENCES

We recommend the use of *Number Needed to Treat* (NNT) and *Number Needed to Harm* (NNH), *Total Number Needed to Harm* (NNH_{Total}) which shows the likelihood for a patient to have at least one adverse effect from using a drug, and *Therapeutic Value* (TV = NNH_{Total}/NNT) (35) which tells us about the balance between beneficial and harmful effects of the drug.

When more objective and reliable data on a pharmaceutical drug exist, i.e. from independent metaanalyses like the Cochrane reviews, they should be preferred before more doubtful data from studies of lower quality, i.e. data from the pharmaceutical industry's own documentation (see table 2).

DISCUSSION

The Swine flu scandal from 2009 showed the world how the present relationship is between the pharmaceutical industry and WHO. During this scandal WHO first declared a fake pandemic followed by recommendations to the WHO member states to spend tens of billions of EUROs and dollars to purchase ineffective and unnecessary influenza vaccines and anti-influenza medicine. The recommendations included two jabs of poorly tested vaccine for every citizen on the planet! During the scandal the media documented a close link between people paid directly by the pharmaceutical companies making the vaccines and the WHO leadership and this was strongly criticized by The European Commission (36), major media, scientific journals, and health authorities in a number of countries (37-68).

The scandal forced WHO to make an investigation of itself which led to the remarkable conclusion that WHO had done nothing wrong: "WHO performed well in many ways during the pandemic…" and "The Committee found no evidence of malfeasance. "(69 p. xvi). With this conclusion WHO has clearly showed the world where it stands: Side by side with the pharmaceutical industry.

With this said it is important to underline that this article do not take the position that drugs cannot be used as medicine. Vaccines have saved millions of humans and there is much good literature to support that. The uses of chemotherapy along with other treatments have lowered the mortality rates for children with leukaemia and other malignancies over the past decades. And if someone is actively hallucinating and hearing voices to kill themselves or others, and has strong urges to follow such voices, antipsychotic medicine might be what is needed here even if this treatment is not improving the patient's mental health i.e. removing the hallucinations.

CONCLUSION

WHO recommends a long list of drugs which in independent meta-analyses Such as the Cochrane Reviews have been found to have little or no value as medicine but often severe adverse effects, including sexual problems, major health problems (i.e., heart problems, sudden death, and even suicide). The recommendations in WHO's drug registers are followed by its 194 member states leading in our estimation to at least 100,000,000 patients getting a wrong treatment. WHO, the organization who was established to solve the health problems of the world, has itself become a major threat to public health worldwide.

We therefore recommend a fundamental revision of the whole WHO-system that has proven itself weak to the interests of the pharmaceutical industry. We warn all governments, physicians, and patients that the existing WHO drug directories are strongly biased and not reliable sources of information on drugs and vaccines. We encourage all WHO member states to use their power as member states to revise the malfunctioning WHO system and set WHO free of the malicious influence of the pharmaceutical industry.

The critique we raise in this article is not new. All financial ties between WHO and the pharmaceutical industry must be cut as Flynn on behalf of the Council of Europe concluded in his famous rapport (36). The funding of WHO should never have been privatized. It simply does not work and was a major mistake. It leads to the corrupted WHO we have today.

In the future all funding of WHO must come from the member states only. The establishment of a new leadership of WHO which can stand the strong and continued pressure from the pharmaceutical industry must be amongst the first action taken; the importance of this action must be acknowledged by WHO's member states. WHO needs urgently new and independent leaders with a strong and well established scientific expertise in the scientific testing of medicine.

ACKNOWLEDGMENTS

The Danish Quality of Life Survey, Quality of Life Research Center and The Research Clinic for Holistic Medicine, Copenhagen, was from 1987 till today supported by grants from the 1991 Pharmacy Foundation, the Goodwill-fonden, the JL-Foundation, E. Danielsen and Wife's Foundation, Emmerick Meyer's Trust, the Frimodt-Heineken Foundation, the Hede Nielsen Family Foundation, Petrus Andersens Fond, Wholesaler C.P. Frederiksens Study Trust, Else & Mogens Wedell-Wedellsborg's Foundation and IMK Almene Fond. The research in quality of life and scientific complementary and holistic medicine was approved by the Copenhagen Scientific Ethical Committee under the numbers (KF) V. 100.1762-90, (KF) V. 100.2123/91, (KF) V. 01-502/93, (KF) V. 01-026/97, (KF) V. 01-162/97, (KF) V. 01-198/97 and further correspondence. We declare no conflict of interest.

Contributorship/transparency statement: This article was done by Søren Ventegodt, who affirms that the manuscript is an honest, accurate, and transparent account of the study being reported; no important aspects of the study have been omitted; any discrepancies from the study as planned have been explained.

REFERENCES

[1] WHO model lists of essential medicines. URL: http://www.who.int/medicines/publications/essentialmedicines/en/index.html

[2] Ventegodt S, Merrick J. A review of the Danish National Drug Directory: Who provides the data for the register? Int J Adolesc Med Health 2010;22(2):197-212.

[3] Abel U. Chemotherapy of advanced epithelial cancer—a critical review. Biomed Pharmacother 1992;46:439-52.

[4] Abel U. [Chemotherapy of advanced epithelial cancer.] Stuttgart: Hippokrates Verlag, 1990. [German]
[5] Abel U. [Chemotherapie fortgesch-rittener Karzi-nome. Eine kritische Bestandsaufnahme.] Berlin: Hippokrates, 1995. [German]
[6] Moncrieff J, Wessely S, Hardy R. Active placebos versus antidepressants for depression. Cochrane Database Syst Rev 2004;1:CD003012.
[7] Adams CE, Awad G, Rathbone J, Thornley B. Chlorpromazine versus placebo for schizophrenia. Cochrane Database Syst Rev 2007;2:CD000284.
[8] Jefferson T, Di Pietrantonj C, Rivetti A, Bawazeer GA, Al-Ansary LA, Ferroni E. Vaccines for preventing influenza in healthy adults. Cochrane Database Syst Rev. 2014 Mar 13;3:CD001269. doi: 10.1002/14651858.CD001269.pub5.
[9] Jefferson T, Jones MA, Doshi P, Del Mar CB, Hama R, Thompson MJ, et al. Neuraminidase inhibitors for preventing and treating influenza in healthy adults and children. Cochrane Database Syst Rev. 2014 Apr 10;4:CD008965. doi: 10.1002/14651858.CD008965.pub4.
[10] Gøtzsche PC. Psychiatry has gone astray. We would be much better off if we took away all psychotropic drugs from the market. The physicians are not able to handle them. [Psykiatri på afveje. Vi ville være langt bedre stillet, hvis alle psykofarmaka blev fjernet fra markedet. Lægerne er ikke i stand til at håndtere dem. Kroniken.] Politiken 2014 Jan 6.
[11] Gøtzsche P. Deadly medicines and organised crime: How big pharma has corrupted healthcare. New York: Radcliffe, 2013.
[12] Gøtzsche PC. Why I think antidepressants cause more harm than good. *Lancet Psychiatry 2014*;1:104-6.
[13] Boutron I, Estellat C, Guittet L, Dechartres A, Sackett DL, Hróbjartsson A, et al. Methods of blinding in reports of randomized controlled trials assessing pharmacologic treatments: a systematic review. PLoS Med 2006;3(10):e425.
[14] Ventegodt S, Andersen NJ, Brom B, Merrick J, Greydanus DE. Evidence-based medicine: Four fundamental problems with the randomised clinical trial (RCT) used to document chemical medicine. Int J Adolesc Med Health 2009;21(4):485-96.
[15] Committee on the Use of Complementary and Alternative Medicine by the American Public. Complementary and Alternative Medicine (CAM) in the United States. Washington, DC: National Academies Press, 2005.
[16] Leichsenring F, Rabung S, Leibing E. The efficacy of short-term psychodynamic psychotherapy in specific psychiatric disorders: a meta-analysis. Arch Gen Psychiatry 2004;61(12):1208-16.
[17] Leichsenring F. Are psychodynamic and psychoanalytic therapies effective? A review of empirical data. Int J Psychoanal 2005;86(Pt 3):841-68.
[18] Leichsenring F, Leibing E. Psychodynamic psychotherapy: a systematic review of techniques, indications and empirical evidence. Psychol Psychother 2007;80(Pt 2):217-28.
[19] Bø K, Berghmans B, Mørkved S, Van Kampen, M. Evidence-based physical physical therapy for the pelvic floor. Bridging science and clinical practice. New York: Elsevier Butterworth Heinemann, 2007.
[20] Sobel DS. Mind matters, money matters: The cost-effectiveness of mind/body medicine. JAMA 2000;284(13):1704.
[21] Astin JA, Shapiro SL, Eisenberg DM, Forys KL. Mindbody medicine: State of the science, implications for practice. J Am Board Fam Pract 2003;16:131-47.
[22] Abbass A, Kisely S, Kroenke K. Short-term psychodynamic psychotherapy for somatic disorders. Systematic review and meta-analysis of clinical trials. Psychother Psychosom 2009;78(5):265-74.
[23] Chopra D, Ornish D , Roy R, Weil A. Alternative' medicine is mainstream. The evidence is mounting that diet and lifestyle are the best cures for our worst afflictions. Wall Street Journal 2009 Jan 9:A13.
[24] Ventegodt S, Merrick J. Textbook on evidence-based holistic mind-body medicine: Basic philosophy and ethics of traditional Hippocratic medicine. New York: Nova Science, 2012.
[25] Ventegodt S, Merrick J. Textbook on evidence-based holistic mind-body medicine: Basic principles of healing in traditional Hippocratic medicine. New York: Nova Science, 2012.
[26] Ventegodt S, Merrick J. Textbook on evidence-based holistic mind-body medicine: Healing the mind in traditional Hippocratic medicine. New York: Nova Science, 2012.

[27] Ventegodt S, Merrick J. Textbook on evidence-based holistic mind-body medicine: Holistic practice of traditional Hippocratic medicine. New York: Nova Science, 2013.
[28] Ventegodt S, Merrick J. Textbook on evidence-based holistic mind-body medicine: Research, philosophy, economy and politics of traditional Hippocratic medicine. New York: Nova Science, 2013.
[29] Ventegodt S, Merrick J. Textbook on evidence-based holistic mind-body medicine: Sexology and traditional Hippocratic medicine. New York: Nova Science, 2013.
[30] Smith R. The drugs don't work. BMJ 2003;327:0-h.
[31] Dansk Cardiologisk Selskab og Dansk Psykiatrisk Selskab. Arytmi-risiko ved anvendelse af psykofarmaka. DCS og DPS vejledning. Copenhagen: Dansk Cardiologisk Selskab og Dansk Psykiatrisk Selskab, 2011;1. [Danish]
[32] Ornish D, Brown SE, Scherwitz LW, Billings JH, Armstrong WT, et al. Can lifestyle changes reverse coronary heart disease? The lifestyle heart trial. Lancet 1990;336(8708):129-33.
[33] Ornish D, Scherwitz LW, Billings JH, Brown SE, Gould KL, et al. Intensive lifestyle changes for reversal of coronary heart disease. JAMA1998;280(23),2001-7.
[34] Frattaroli J, Weidner G, Dnistrian AM, Kemp C, Daubenmier JJ, Marlin RO, et al. Clinical events in prostate cancer lifestyle trial: results from two years of follow-up. Urology 2008;72(6):1319-23.
[35] Ventegodt S, Merrick J. Therapeutic value (TV) of treatments with pharmaceutical drugs. Rough estimates for all clinical conditions based on Cochrane reviews and the ratio: Number Needed to Harm/Number Needed to Treat (TV=NNH$_{total}$/NNT). BMJ 2010 Nov 15. URL: http://www.bmj.com/content/341/bmj.c5715.full/reply#bmj_el_244738
[36] Council of Europe and Flynn P. The handling of the H1N1 pandemic: more transparency needed. 4 June 2010. URL: *assembly.coe.int/CommitteeDocs/2010/20100604_H1N1pandemic_E.pdf*
[37] ABC news. World Health Organization Scientists Linked to Swine Flu Vaccine Makers, 2010 Jun 5. URL: http://abcnews.go.com/Health/SwineFlu/swine-flu-pandemic-world-health-organization-scientists-linked/story?id=10829940
[38] BBC. Way opened for Pandemrix swine flu jab compensation. Bbc.com, 2013 Sept 20. URL: http://www.bbc.com/news/health-24172715
[39] BBC. WHO swine flu experts 'linked' with drug companies, 2010 Jan 4. URL: http://www.bbc.com/news/10235558
[40] Bethge P, Elger K, Glüsing J, Grill M, Hachenbroch V, Puhl J, et al. Reconstruction of a Mass Hysteria: The Swine Flu Panic of 2009. Der Spiegel 2010 Mar 12. Part 1. URL: http://www.spiegel.de/international/world/reconstruction-of-a-mass-hysteria-the-swine-flu-panic-of-2009-a-682613.html
[41] Bethge P, Elger K, Glüsing J, Grill M, Hachenbroch V, Puhl J, et al. Reconstruction of a Mass Hysteria: The Swine Flu Panic of 2009. Der Spiegel 2010 Mar 12. Part 2. URL: http://www.spiegel.de/international/world/reconstruction-of-a-mass-hysteria-the-swine-flu-panic-of-2009-a-682613-2.html
[42] Braillon A. The World Health Organization: no game of thrones. BMJ 2014 Jun 26. URL: http://www.bmj.com/content/348/bmj.g4265/rr/703675
[43] Cohen D, Carter P. Key scientists advising the World Health Organization on planning for an influenza pandemic had done paid work for pharmaceutical firms that stood to gain from the guidance they were preparing. These conflicts of interest have never been publicly disclosed by WHO, and WHO has dismissed inquiries into its handling of the A/H1N1 pandemic as "conspiracy theories." BMJ 2010;340:c2912. URL: http://www.bmj.com/content/340/bmj.c2912
[44] Cohen D, Carter P. Conflicts of interest. WHO and the pandemic flu "conspiracies." BMJ 2010;340:c2912. doi: 10.1136/bmj.c2912. No abstract available.
[45] Cohen D, Carter P. WHO and the pandemic flu "conspiracies". BMJ 2009 Jun 4. URL: http://www.bmj.com/content/340/bmj.c2912
[46] Doshi P, Jefferson T. WHO and pandemic flu. Another question for GSK. BMJ 2010;340:c3455. doi: 10.1136/bmj.c3455.
[47] Editorial. Report condemns swine flu experts' ties to big pharma. The Guardian 2010 Jun 4. URL: http://www.theguardian.com/business/2010/jun/04/swine-flu-experts-big-pharmaceutical

[48] Editorial. Australian journalist wins prestigious award for exposing flu vaccine scandal. The Refusers 2011 Novr 28. URL: http://therefusers.com/refusers-newsroom/australian-journalist-wins-prestigious-award-for-exposing-flu-vaccine-scandal/
[49] Edwards T. Big pharma probed for 'false' swine flu pandemic. The Week 2010 Jan 11. URL: http://www.theweek.co.uk/politics/17419/big-pharma-probed-%E2%80%98false%E2%80%99-swine-flu-pandemic
[50] Ejbye AE, Korsgaard P. Only one out of 100 is helped by the flu vaccine. [Kun en ud af 100 har gavn af influenzavaccine.] Ekstra Bladet 2013 Dec 22. URL: http://ekstrabladet.dk/kup/ sundhed/article 4620514.ece
[51] Fletcher V. Swine flu scandal: Billions of pounds are wasted on vaccines. Express 2014 Nov 12. URL: http://www.express.co.uk/news/uk/156359/Swine-flu-scandal-Billions-
[52] Fletcher V. Swine flu scandal: Billions of pounds are wasted on vaccines. Express 2014 Oct 27. URL: http://www.express.co.uk/news/uk/156359/Swine-flu-scandal-Billions-of-pounds-are-wasted-on-vaccines
[53] Galushko I. The reality behind the swine flu conspiracy. RT 2009 Dec 5. URL: http://rt.com/politics/reality-swine-flu-conspiracy/
[54] Information. Can we trust the WHO? [Tør vi stole på WHO?] Information 2009 Dec 12. URL: http://www.information.dk/218357
[55] Interview with Epidemiologist Tom Jefferson. A whole industry is waiting for a pandemic. The world has been gripped with fears of swine flu in recent weeks. In an interview with SPIEGEL, epidemiologist Tom Jefferson speaks about dangerous fear-mongering, misguided, money-driven research and why we should all be washing our hands a lot more often. Der Spiegel 2009 Jul 21.
[56] Jefferson T, Doshi P. WHO and pandemic flu. Time for change, WHO. BMJ 2010;340:c3461. URL: http://www.bmj.com/cgi/content/extract/340/jun29_4/c3461
[57] JeffersonT, Doshi P. Multisystem failure: the story of anti-influenza drugs. BMJ 2014 Apr 10. URL: http://www.bmj.com/content/348/bmj.g2263
[58] Law R. WHO and pandemic flu. There was also no new subtype. BMJ 2010;340:c3460. doi: 10.1136/bmj.c3460.
[59] Neale T. World Health Organization scientists linked to swine flu vaccine makers. ABC News 2010 Jun 5. URL: http://abcnews.go.com/Health/SwineFlu/swine-flu-pandemic-world-health-organization-scientists-linked/story?id=10829940
[60] Payne D. Tamiflu: The battle for secret drug data. BMJ 2012 Oct 29. URL: http://www.bmj.com/content/345/bmj.e7303
[61] Hodler R, Loertscher S, Rohner D. Biased experts, costly lies, and binary decisions. ResearchGate 2010. URL: http://www.researchgate.net/publication/46476997_Biased_experts_co
[62] Sample I. Swine flu vaccine can trigger narcolepsy, UK government concedes. The Guardian 2013 Sept 19. URL: http://www.theguardian.com/society/2013/sep/19/swine-flu-vaccine-narcolepsy-uk
[63] Shanahan C. Law firm not expecting swine flu narcolepsy case in court before 2016. Irish Examiner 2014 Sept 15. URL: http://www.irishexaminer.com/ireland/law-firm-not-expecting-swine-flu-narcolepsy-case-in-court-before-2016-286331.html
[64] Sørensen A. Vaccine has serious adverse effects [Vaccine forbindes med alvorlige bivirkninger.] Berlinske 2009 Nov 14. URL: http://www.b.dk/danmark/vaccine-forbindes-med-alvorlige-bivirkninger
[65] Sørensen AB, Cuculiza M. Influenza vaccine: The health authorities are hiding serious adverse effects [Influenzavaccine: Sundhedsstyrelsen fortier alvorlige bivirkninger.] MX 2014 Oct 20. URL: http://www.mx.dk/nyheder/danmark/story/22774533
[66] Stein R. Reports accuse WHO of exaggerating H1N1 threat, possible ties to drug makers. Washington Post 2010 Jun 4. URL: http://www.washingtonpost.com/wp-dyn/content/article/2010/06/04/AR2010060403034.html
[67] Watson R. WHO is accused of "crying wolf" over swine flu pandemic. BMJ 2010;340:c1904. doi: 10.1136/bmj.c1904.

[68] Zarocostas J. Swine flu pandemic review panel seeks access to confidential documents between WHO and drug companies. BMJ 2010;340:c2792. doi: 10.1136/bmj.c2792.
[69] World Health Organization: Report of the strengthening response to pandemics and other public-health emergencies. Report of the review committee on the functioning of the international health regulations (2005) and on pandemic influenza (h1n1) 2009. Geneva: WHO, 2012.

In: Mental and Holistic Health: Some International Perspectives   ISBN: 978-1-63483-589-3
Editors: J. Calles Jr., D. Greydanus and J. Merrick   © 2015 Nova Science Publishers, Inc.

Chapter 10

ALTERNATIVE MEDICINE (NON-DRUG MEDICINE, CAM) VERSUS PHARMACOLOGICAL MEDICINE

Søren Ventegodt[*], MD, MMedSci, EU-MSc-CAM

Quality of Life Research Center, Copenhagen, Denmark,
Research Clinic for Holistic Medicine and Nordic School of Holistic Medicine,
Copenhagen, Denmark

ABSTRACT

In evidence-based medicine you need to look at the quality of the scientific evidence. The best scientific evidence, like the metaanalyses made by independent researchers like the Cochrane reviews has systematically shown that some drugs are of little help for patients and even harmful. Is complementary and alternative medicine (CAM) effective? A number of scientific studies of prayers and positive thinking, diets, exercises, breathing exercises, yoga, meditation, art therapy, herbal medicine and more, have proven these types of CAM to be without significant positive effect for the patient. Therefore, in general, CAM cures are not working. With this said there are some types of talk and touch therapy that has been proven extremely effective. That is the methods that at the same time focus on 1) feelings and emotions including sexuality, 2) understanding and self-exploration including almost all types of self-inquiry, and 3) letting go of negative beliefs, attitudes, thoughts, philosophies and concepts. The true problem of therapy is that some people just seem to have what it takes to become a therapist; they are good from the beginning of their practice even without education and training. Everybody can heal, everybody can become happy. But to heal from a serious disease we need to change from a very deep place within ourselves. Facilitating this inner change that in the end will transform our whole being and experience of life is what all effective medicine is about.

---

[*] Correspondence: Søren Ventegodt, MD, MMedSci, EUMSc-CAM, Director, Quality of Life Research Center, Frederiksberg Alle 13A, 2tv, DK-1661 Copenhagen V, Denmark. E-mail: ventegodt@livskvalitet.org

INTRODUCTION

Good scientific medicine has two major components: It has good theory and it has good clinical documentation.

Human beings are bio-psycho-social beings (1); while science is quite clear and simple when it comes to chemistry, physics and biology, it gets quite unclear and flimsy when it comes to psychology, and really messy when it comes to the social dimensions of mankind.

Good medicine theory is interdisciplinary; it describes man as a bio-psycho-social being and disease as a disturbance in the wholeness, not in one of its parts. When you get sick, the symptoms are often in your body, but the cause is in your psyche; and if you explore your mental dimension you will find that it is highly dependent on you social reality.

If you look at the immune system its immunological defense power comes from the inner balance of the organism (2); but this balance is hard to describe in scientific terms. We know that staying healthy is closely related to quality of life and happiness; you can say that happiness is the best medicine.

The biological and cellular order is highly sensitive to the state of mind of the person; but happiness goes even deeper. Happiness goes to the roots of you being and stretches out to the most remote of your relationships. Your happiness vibrates though you whole existence. Happiness is a mystery in itself; there is no really good science about happiness, so to include happiness in the scientific theory of medicine has been and remains a real challenge. This work has simply not been done yet. We have a lot of research to do here in the future! What we can say for sure is that a simple chemical model for life is totally inadequate to explain health, disease, bad thriving, and healing.

SCIENTIFIC DOCUMENTATION

When it comes to scientific documentation of the clinical effect of medicine, we have even bigger problems, for what is a good test of clinical effect? We know by now that the randomized clinical trial (RCT), which everybody 30 years ago believed to be the final solution to the problem of how to test pharmacological medicine is so faulty and flawed that it cannot be taken as scientific documentation (3).

One problem is that the active placebo effect of poisonous drugs in the RCT-test, as it is designed today, turns all poisonous drugs tested by the method into effective medicine with exactly the specific action the test aims to explore (3,4). This is a hopeless situation; the blinding is always broken by the toxic effects of the drugs and the pharmaceutical companies are producing "medicines", which have toxic effects (3-5). A number of Cochrane studies have recently documented that many of the drug-groups we are using are without significant beneficial effects, but poisonous (5, 6). Yet 100 million people or so are taking these drugs every day in the belief that they are helpful. And because of the active placebo they are helpful for a short while. But this is like peeing your pants to get heat: It only helps for a very short time; then it gets really annoying.

The consequence of the lack of a valid test method for pharmacological drugs has been devastating; According to leading experts in the Cochrane Collaboration millions of patients are getting "poisoned" with severe consequences for their health every year; and thousands of these patients are even dying from the poisoning (5). Especially the psychiatric patients are burdened by the toxic effects of the drugs (6).

EVIDENCE-BASED MEDICINE

In evidence-based medicine you need to look at the quality of the scientific evidence. The best scientific evidence, like the metaanalyses made by independent researchers i.e. the Cochrane reviews from the 3,000 fairly independent physicians and researchers in the international Cochrane collaboration, has systematically shown that some drugs are of little help for patients and even harmful. Even the best of pharmacological medicines has surprisingly little effect; if you look at how many patients you need to treat for one being helped (the NNT number) it is normally 20 patients or more (7) (and often 100 or more for serious diseases like cancer and schizophrenia).

An NNT of 20 means that if a doctor gives such a drug to a patient, the likelihood for the patient to be helped is 0.05, or only 5%! If NNT = 100 only 1% of the patients are helped. And the people who are helped are most often NOT cured. They only have little less symptoms of the disease. So this is the situation of the pharmacological medicine we have today. At the same time, adverse effects are so normal that on average every patient will have a harmful effect from taking a drug (8). Honestly it is not worth being a doctor with such poor results. Therefore many doctors burn out and loose the joy of work while they year after year see that their patients systematically are not improving.

So how is it with evidence-based CAM – alternative medicine, non-drug medicine - call it what you like? Today hundreds of metaanalyses and Cochrane reviews have shown that there are no significant side effects of non-drug medicine (9, 10) with high-energy manipulations (chiropractic) as a rare exception. So you can safely go to any psychotherapist or body worker. Talk and touch therapy are just safe (10). That is good to know.

ALTERNATIVE MEDICINE

But is CAM effective? Well, in general alternative medicine is not effective. Sorry. If you look at all that we do to help and cure, this broad spectrum of activities we call CAM are mostly NOT helpful. A number of scientific studies of prayers and positive thinking, diets, exercises, breathing exercises, yoga, meditation, art therapy, herbal medicine and more, have proven these types of CAM to be without significant positive effect for the patient (9). Therefore, in general, CAM cures are not working.

With this said there are some types of talk and touch therapy that has been proven extremely effective. That is the methods that at the same time focus on 1) feelings and emotions including sexuality, 2) understanding and self-exploration including almost all types of self-inquiry, and 3) letting go of negative beliefs, attitudes, thoughts, philosophies, concepts etc. – i.e., mind-work that empties your mind from all its mental contents and structures, and all our identifications (11-16).

Psychodynamic psychotherapy – i.e., talk therapy with focus on emotions and sexuality – have been proven extremely effective; 95% have been helped and the help is often a cure (17-

19). Holistic medicine has recently in the USA been found extremely effective for cancer and coronary heart disease, with 80% of the patients or so helped within 3-6 month (20-22). These are amazing results.

Similar results have been found for a number of existentially oriented talk-and touch therapies (23, 24). Methods that combine talk and touch therapy to help the patient FEEL, UNDERSTAND and LET GO of negative beliefs have in general been found very effective, with amazing NNT numbers [1 or 2] and totally harmless. And the wonderful thing is that these methods seem to help a wide range of clinical conditions – almost all types of patients can be helped (25). And these results are also found in metaanalyses made by independent researchers. See, this is good, evidence-based medicine. So we have after all come a long way in medicine.

The true problem of therapy is that some people just seem to have what it takes to become a therapist; they are good from the beginning of their practice even without education and training and they become only a little better as years go by (26). And then there is the other group of therapists; the hardworking people with good intentions and little talent who will do much, but accomplish little (27).

IT IS ALL ABOUT LOVE

As we have not been able to teach these therapists how to become good therapists we obviously do not understand what it is that makes a good therapist. In my experience it is about love. Some people simply love other people. These people can help almost everybody – because of their love as Martin Buber (1878-1965) pointed out (28). They don't judge; they don't create a distance to their clients or patients. They just accept, acknowledge, care, and support whoever comes to them (29).

You cannot learn to love. If you do not love other people, you cannot be trained to do so. So in the end of the day, it all comes down to this simple thing: if you want to be a therapist ask if you love other people. If you don't and you still want to become therapist you might want to look at your motives. Being a bad therapist will not serve the world. But if you love other people just start today and open your practice. You will without doubt succeed.

Maybe you will wonder how these things fit together: That some methods seem to work, but that people cannot learn therapy. It seems that people with a talent for therapy are simply attracted to effective methods that focus on important issues like the meaning of life (30).

It takes a lot of love to work with people's feelings and sexuality; to help the sick and insane to explore there innermost secrets and to work patiently endless numbers of hours to help neurotic people to let go of untrue believes (27).

If you are troubled and in search for a good therapist yourself, don't waste your time reading science. Go and look for somebody who can love and serve you. Find a therapist with whom you have a good chemistry, a person you can feel you can trust and love yourself. If you can find such a person this is you best change for getting the help you need to change your life.

Everybody can heal, everybody can become happy. But to heal from a serious disease we need to change from a very deep place within ourselves. Facilitating this inner change that in the end will transform our whole being and experience of life is what all effective medicine is about (31).

ACKNOWLEDGMENTS

The Danish Quality of Life Survey, Quality of Life Research Center and The Research Clinic for Holistic Medicine, Copenhagen, was from 1987 till today supported by grants from the 1991 Pharmacy Foundation, the Goodwill-fonden, the JL-Foundation, E. Danielsen and Wife's Foundation, Emmerick Meyer's Trust, the Frimodt-Heineken Foundation, the Hede Nielsen Family Foundation, Petrus Andersens Fond, Wholesaler C.P. Frederiksens Study Trust, Else & Mogens Wedell-Wedellsborg's Foundation and IMK Almene Fond. The research in quality of life and scientific complementary and holistic medicine was approved by the Copenhagen Scientific Ethical Committee under the numbers (KF) V. 100.1762-90, (KF) V. 100.2123/91, (KF) V. 01-502/93, (KF) V. 01-026/97, (KF)V. 01-162/97, (KF)V. 01-198/97 and further correspondence. We declare no conflict of interest.

REFERENCES

[1] Ventegodt S, Flensborg-Madsen T, Andersen NJ, Nielsen M, Morad M, Merrick J. Global quality of life (QOL), health and ability are primarily determined by our consciousness. Research findings from Denmark 1991-2004. Soc Indicat Res 2005;71;87-122.

[2] Ventegodt S, Omar H, Merrick J. Quality of life as medicine: Interventions that induce salutogenesis. A review of the literature. Soc Indicat Res 2011;100(3):415-33.

[3] Ventegodt S, Andersen NJ, Brom B, Merrick J, Greydanus DE. Evidence-based medicine: Four fundamental problems with the randomised clinical trial (RCT) used to document chemical medicine. Int J Adolesc Med Health 2009;21(4):485-96.

[4] Boutron I, Estellat C, Guittet L, Dechartres A, Sackett DL, Hrobjartsson A, Ravaud P. Methods of blinding in reports of randomized controlled trials assessing pharmacologic treatments: A systematic review. PLoS Med 2006;3(10):e425.

[5] Gøtzsche P. Deadly medicines and organised crime: How big pharma has corrupted healthcare". New York: Radcliffe, 2013.

[6] 6. Gøtzsche PC. Psychiatry has gone astray. We would be much better off if we took away all psychotropic drugs from the market. The physicians are not able to handle them. [Psykiatri på afveje. Vi ville være langt bedre stillet, hvis alle psykofarmaka blev fjernet fra markedet. Lægerne er ikke i stand til at håndtere dem]. Politiken 2014 Jan 6. [Danish]

[7] Smith R. The drugs don't work. BMJ 2003;327(7428):0-h.

[8] Ventegodt S, Merrick J. Therapeutic value (TV) of treatments with pharmaceutical drugs. Rough estimates for all clinical conditions based on Cochrane reviews and the ratio: Number Needed to Harm/Number Needed to Treat (TV=NNHtotal/NNT). BMJ, Nov 15, 2010. http://www.bmj.com/content/341/bmj.c5715.full/reply#bmj_el_244738

[9] Committee on the Use of Complementary and Alternative Medicine by the American Public. Complementary and Alternative Medicine (CAM) in the United States. Washington, DC: National Academies Press, 2005.

[10] Ventegodt S, Merrick J. A review of side effects and adverse events of non-drug medicine (nonpharmaceutical complementary and alternative medicine): Psychotherapy, mind-body medicine and clinical holistic medicine. J Complement Integr Med 2009;6(1):16.

[11] Ventegodt S, Merrick J. Textbook on evidence-based holistic mind-body medicine: Basic philosophy and ethics of traditional Hippocratic medicine. New York: Nova Science, 2012.
[12] Ventegodt S, Merrick J. Textbook on evidence-based holistic mind-body medicine: Basic principles of healing in traditional Hippocratic medicine. New York: Nova Science, 2012.
[13] Ventegodt S, Merrick J. Textbook on evidence-based holistic mind-body medicine: Healing the mind in traditional Hippocratic medicine. New York: Nova Science, 2012.
[14] Ventegodt S, Merrick J. Textbook on evidence-based holistic mind-body medicine: Holistic practice of traditional Hippocratic medicine. New York: Nova Science, 2013.
[15] Ventegodt S, Merrick J. Textbook on evidence-based holistic mind-body medicine: Research, philosophy, economy and politics of traditional Hippocratic medicine. New York: Nova Science, 2013.
[16] Ventegodt S, Merrick J. Textbook on evidence-based holistic mind-body medicine: Sexology and traditional Hippocratic Medicine. New York: Nova Science, 2013.
[17] Leichsenring F, Rabung S, Leibing E. The efficacy of short-term psychodynamic psychotherapy in specific psychiatric disorders: a meta-analysis. Arch Gen Psychiatry 2004;61(12):1208-16.
[18] Leichsenring F. Are psychodynamic and psychoanalytic therapies effective? A review of empirical data. Int J Psychoanal 2005;86(Pt 3):841-68.
[19] Leichsenring F, Leibing E. Psychodynamic psychotherapy: a systematic review of techniques, indications and empirical evidence. Psychol Psychother 2007;80(Pt 2):217-28.
[20] Ornish D, Brown SE, Scherwitz LW, Billings JH, Armstrong WT, et al. Can lifestyle changes reverse coronary heart disease? The lifestyle heart trial. Lancet 1990;336(8708):129-33.
[21] Ornish D, Scherwitz LW, Billings JH, Brown SE, Gould KL, et al. Intensive lifestyle changes for reversal of coronary heart disease. JAMA 1998;280(23):2001-7.
[22] Frattaroli J, Weidner G, Dnistrian AM, Kemp C, Daubenmier JJ, Marlin RO, et al. Clinical events in prostate cancer lifestyle trial: results from two years of follow-up. Urology 2008;72(6):1319-23.
[23] Allmer C, Ventegodt S, Kandel I, Merrick J. Positive effects, side effects, and adverse events of clinical holistic medicine. A review of Gerda Boyesen's nonpharmaceutical mind-body medicine (biodynamic body-psychotherapy) at two centers in the United Kingdom and Germany. Int J Adolesc Med Health. 2009;21(3):281-97.
[24] Ventegodt S, Merrick J. Meta-analysis of positive effects, side effects and adverse events of holistic mind-body medicine (clinical holistic medicine): experience from Denmark, Sweden, United Kingdom and Germany. Int J Adolesc Med Health 2009;21(4):441-56.
[25] Ventegodt S, Andersen NJ, Kandel I, Merrick J. Comparative analysis of cost-effectiveness of non-drug medicine (non-pharmaceutical holistic, complementary and alternative medicine/CAM) and biomedicine (pharmaceutical drugs) for all clinical conditions. Int J Disabil Hum Dev 2009;8(3):245-56.
[26] Goleman D. Healing emotions: Conversations with the Dalai Lama on the mindfulness, emotions, and health. Boston, MA: Mind Life Institute, 1997.
[27] Kierkegaard SA. The sickness unto death. Princeton, NJ: Princeton University Press, 1983.
[28] Buber M. I and thou. New York: Charles Scribner, 1970.
[29] Maslow AH. Toward a psychology of being, New York: Van Nostrand,1962.
[30] Frankl V. Man´s search for meaning. New York: Pocket Books, 1985.
[31] Antonovsky A. Unravelling the mystery of health. How people manage stress and stay well. San Francisco, CA: Jossey-Bass, 1987.

In: Mental and Holistic Health: Some International Perspectives   ISBN: 978-1-63483-589-3
Editors: J. Calles Jr., D. Greydanus and J. Merrick   © 2015 Nova Science Publishers, Inc.

Chapter 11

MEDICAL USE OF THE HALLUCINOGENIC TEA AYAHUASCA IN PERU

Søren Ventegodt, MD, MMedSci, EU-MSc-CAM[1,2,3,4,*] and Pavlina Kordova[1,2,3]

[1]Quality of Life Research Center, Copenhagen, Denmark
[2]Research Clinic for Holistic Medicine, Copenhagen, Denmark
[3]Nordic School of Holistic Medicine, Copenhagen, Denmark
[4]Scandinavian Foundation for Holistic Medicine, Sandvika, Norway

ABSTRACT

The use of hallucinogens as medicine has a long history as this was the dominant form of medicine in most premodern cultures. We have studied premodern medicine on the different continents and have been surprised over the level of knowledge and understanding we found in Peru, where the shamans, the Ayahuasqueros, seem to have an extraordinary high level of mastery of the use of hallucinogenic drugs as medicine. Ayahuasca, a mixture of two plants found in the jungle, has the hallucinogenic power similar to LSD-25, and because of an ingenuous pharmacological system its effect last as long as LSD, or even longer. We spent a month in Peru and travelled more than 1,500 km through the north of Peru and the Peruvian Amazonia in the attempt to find the most rational, safe and effective way to use Ayahuasca as medicine. We are content to report that a system with five consecutive days of Ayahuasca, supported by an Ayahuasquero trained in philosophy of life, allowed the patient to go deeper into the unconscious every day, followed by five days of silent reflection and contemplation is an extremely effective scheme for healing and possible the best way of using hallucinogens as medicine. It seems rational to use 150-500 µg LSD-25 in clinical research with hallucinogens as medicine as the dose and duration of the session seems to be difficult even for a trained shaman to control, when using Ayahuasca.

---

[*] Correspondence: Søren Ventegodt, MD, MMedSci, EUMSc-CAM, Director, Quality of Life Research Center, Fredriksberg Alle 13A, 2tv, DK-1661 Copenhagen V, Denmark. E-mail: ventegodt@livskvalitet.org

INTRODUCTION

Ayahuasca, also commonly called yagé, is a mixture of the liana Ayahuasca (which refers to a number of wine species including Banisteriopsis caapi) containing a MAO-inhibitor and Chacruna (shrubs of the genus Psychotria), which contains DMT (N,N-Dimethyltryptamine). It has been used as medicine for all kinds of mental and physical diseases by Native Americans of the Amazon Jungle and adjacent regions for at least 5000 years (1-9).

Today Ayahuasca seems to be used by almost all tribes in the Amazon Jungle and also by shamans in a large area of South America geographically connected to the jungle. The shamans grow the plants, harvest them in the jungle or import them from herb collectors from the Amazonas. Ayahuasca is legal in Peru and many doctors, psychologists, therapists, and philosophers are giving Ayahuasca to their patients and clients, for healing, existential learning, personal development and spiritual transformation.

Ayahuasca is strongly hallucinogenic and a normal dose has the hallucinogenic effect similar to 150-250μg LSD-25, while a big dose corresponds to 500 μg LSD-25. The effect is normally believed to be the cerebral effect of DMT, protected from catabolism in the digestive system by the MAO-inhibitor in the potion. The Ayahuasca tea can provoke vomiting and diarrhoea, but is known from thousand years of use by the natives not to have any serious adverse effects. It is noteworthy that Ayahuasca can be taken many days in a row without giving the symptoms of exhaustion and tiring that normally follows the use of strong hallucinogens like mescaline, LSD and psilocybin. The shamanistic way is to use Ayahuasca in a sacred ritual for purification, healing and enlightenment. Many modern therapists do not consider the ritual important and put the main emphasis on physical aspects like the diet following the treatment.

OUR VISIT

We travelled for a month through the northern parts of Peru, following a 1,500 km long route from Lima to Huanchaco, further to Tarapoto, then to Pucallpa, Huanuco, Huancayo, and finally back to Lima. Our aim was to study the different ways Ayahuasca is used today, to establish the most beneficial, efficient and rational way to use Ayahuasca and similar hallucinogens in medicine. Our strategy was to combine our knowledge from studies in holistic medicine with personal experience by participating in Ayahuasca treatments.

We soon learned that the use of Ayahuasca varied so much that it did not have any meaning to try all the different strategies. Some Ayahuasqueros treat their patients with Ayahuasca every day many days in a row; others every second day, others again one a week, month or year. Some Ayahuasqueros put their clients on an extremely strict diet weeks or even months before and after the treatment, while others put much less emphasis on the diet. Some Ayahuasqueros gave Ayahuasca to everybody who could pay, while others were very careful in the selection of the clients, so only the "fitted" was accepted into the treatment.

With this wide spectrum of different uses, strategies and intentions behind the ceremony, we had to start by understanding the process of healing by participating in an Ayahuasca ritual ourselves. Having some basic experience we felt more competent to analyse the large number of different and diverse treatment strategies. We found these in the literature, on the internet, and finally by interviews with Ayahuasqueros we met while travelling in Peru. In the end we found what we believe is a rational method for using Ayahuasca for healing; we accepted to personally engage in the healing project, to confirm or falsify our conclusion, that this was an effective and rational way to use Ayahuasca.

AYAHUASCA PHARMACOLOGY

A PubMed search for "Ayahuasca" gave 164 papers (June 2015), showing a good understanding of the psychopharmacology of Ayahuasca, but only a moderate scientific interest in the many possibilities of using Ayahuasca for healing diseases documented in single case rapports (10-43).

DMT or N,N-Dimethyltryptamine was first obtained as a synthetic product by Manske in 1931, when it was isolated as the N-oxide from the seeds of Anadenanthera peregrine, the putative source of a Piaroa psychotropic snuff. Today, DMT is known to occur in over fifty plant species and to be a major active component of Ayahuasca and other psychotropic plant preparations.

DMT appears to fit the characteristics of the so-called psychedelic or hallucinogenic drugs, which share the following characteristics regarding their human pharmacology: 1) modifications in thought processes, perception and mood predominate over other alterations; 2) intellectual capacity and memory is minimally affected or enhanced; 3) stupor, narcosis or excessive stimulation are not the predominant effects; 4) autonomic side effects are moderate and 5) addictive craving is minimal.

The classification of DMT into this pharmacological group is further supported by its chemical structure, and its receptor affinity profile, since the "classical hallucinogens" are agents that: a) bind at 5-HT2 serotonin receptors, and b) are recognized by animals trained to discriminate 1-(2,5-dimethoxy-4-methylphenyl)-2-aminopropane (DOM) from vehicle" - two additional criteria which DMT has been demonstrated to meet.

The ingenious combination of the Ayahuasca liana, containing mono amine oxidase-inhibitors and Chacruna containing the DMT allows the DMT of the final mixture, the Ayahuasca tea, to reach the blood stream and hence the brain, as it passes freely over the blood-brain barrier. The slow release of DMT gives the trip its exceptionally long duration, which is an important feature in the healing process.

THE PERUVIAN AYAHUASCA SCENE:
CHOOSING OUR AYAHUASQUERO

Since there is such a wide range of Shamans and Ayahuasqueros it is of extreme importance who you choose to guide you. Ayahuasqueros varies from the many illiterate street sellers that offer you a mixture of jewels and nice handcraft, magical amulets and Ayahuasca trips, to the expensive western-style medical clinics, who offers Ayahuasca treatment primarily to American tourists and further to the really competent and serious well-studied and well-reflected Ayahuasqueros who are trained in the tradition of the Amazon Ayahuasqueros, and who proudly carries this thousand year old tradition.

In our search for the optimal way to use Ayahuasca as medicine we avoided Ayahuasqueros – and they came in hundreds - who seem to be incompetent and only involved in Ayahuasca to make money. We also avoided the western-style medical clinics that use Ayahuasca without the wisdom of the native Americans, in the belief that it is the drug itself that heals, and not the healing ritual in its totality, allowing the patient to dive into the deep philosophy of life and understanding of purification, healing and personal growth that are behind the traditional shamanistic healing.

We focused on the shamans who regarded Ayahuasca as a mix of mind-expanding teacher plants that take the patients into healing states of consciousness. Teacher plant is how Ayahuasca is often called by natives.

After travelling for weeks without finding what we regarded as a really competent Ayahuasquero, we were one evening searching for Ayahuasqueros on the internet, and here we found Shaman Ronald Rivera Cachique from Pucallpa. A few hours later we were on a small airplane flying from Tarapoto to Pucallpa. We were invited to a personal meeting with Ronald who questioned our intentions. We were finally accepted for an Ayahuasca ceremony, and the Shaman suggested that he could make a ritual in his place in the jungle just for two of us without any other participants. We gratefully accepted his offer.

We were told that the effect of Ayahuasca varied from individual to individual. Some problems can be healed in a week, while other problems need more time. The ritual should take eleven days. The first day we had to accept a tobacco ceremony aimed for our purification as a preparation for the Ayahuasca ceremony. After this we had Ayahuasca for five days in a row. After this we had five days of deep contemplation and healing, resting in peace and doing nothing. We agreed to pay 600 USD including transportation, full accommodation in double room, simple food and the tobacco and the Ayahuasca rituals. The diet started immediately and lasted for all in all 11 days. The ritual then took place in a primitive jungle settlement a two hour drive on very bad jungle roads and about 30 km from Pucallpa.

RONALD RIVERA CACHIQUE ON THE SACRED MEDICINE AYAHUASCA

We were attracted to Ronald, the author of several books on philosophy of life and Ayahuasca, because of his presentation on the internet, which here is repeated in a short form.

Ayahuasca is a ritual medicine used by Amazon healers for thousands of years. It has medicinal benefits for the body and the mind; it allows the awakening of the existential sense and the development of the mystic self. Ayahuasca is always drunk in the context of a ritual medicine, to reaffirm convictions, to contact the mythical world, to acquire valour, to cultivate personal wisdom and to shed light on the future.

Etymologically, Ayahuasca is a Quechua word that signifies: Aya = death or spirit and Huasca = rope or vine. It is translated as: rope of the dead, vine of the soul, climbing plant of the souls or vine that brings us to the world of the gods. The etymological notion synchronizes perfectly with the concept of the enthneogenic plant, a term which some contemporary scholars of this theme use to refer to those substances that have the ability to bring God alive within oneself.

Closely linked to the notion of the Sacred Plant, is the concept of Ayahuasca as a Teacher Plant which, strictly speaking, is not an exaggeration or a superstition, because the experience with Ayahuasca actually does produce a bounty of a personal wisdom. The extraordinary state of consciousness that Ayahuasca produces is a fount of revelation, inspiration and awareness. Ayahuasca creates an awakening of consciousness, a spiritual initiation, and an evolution or personal development.

This initiation is a strong awakening of consciousness. It is an entrance into the spiritual world. It is a renewal of physical and mental energies. It is an evolution of our way of seeing and understanding things. It is enrichment and strengthening of our cosmovision. The initiation with Ayahuasca is the capturing of the real meaning of our existence. Therefore, Ayahuasca is a sacred medicine. That is to say, it produces medicinal effects to help the body and the mind and to inspire the awakening of a personal mysticism. Both aspects, the healing or revitalization and the spiritual realization, notably improve the state of health, both physical and mental, of the participants in Ayahuasca rituals. Of course, the achievement of the benefits or learning necessarily implies a discipline, a process of sensitivity and communication with the spirit of the plants.

It is important to understand that Ayahuasca is a very special medicine that must be drunk in a ritual context, with great respect and under the supervision or assistance of a master Ayahuasquero who is serious and experienced.

It is common for a healer or shaman to be seen as a folkloric person, arrested in the past, and always offering an ethnic and exotic spectacle. The shamanic profile has been caricaturized too much and shamanism reduced to a folkloric and laughable activity. In many societies, the shaman is associated with charlatanism, with fraud and with scams. We must distinguish well between the practice of honest healing with Ayahuasca and the unscrupulous actions of supposed "healers" or "shamans" that sully the traditional medicine. The shamanic fraud is devoid of what is fundamental, that is, the extraordinary state of consciousness that Ayahuasca produces and its most important benefit, the awakening of consciousness. Therefore, the quack "healers" do not promote self-discovery or the expansion of consciousness. With this deceit or transgression, the unscrupulous "Ayahuasqueros" are undermining Ayahuasca, assembling an entire shamanic paraphernalia and choreography to lure the tourists who are hungry for exotic and mystical experiences. Without preparation or deep insight, these makeshift people venture to conduct alleged sessions that end in the violation of women, robberies and in unfortunate psychological consequences, such as psychotic depression and mental confusion.

Ayahuasca is not a tourist attraction that can be offered to every traveller, as one would offer a pisco sour. The experience of drinking Ayahuasca requires a commitment and a very serious discipline. It is not something that can be drunk in passing, later to return to your usual habits. Participants must be selected and prequalified; it is not for everyone.

Among those who do not understand, it is said that Ayahuasca is a hallucinogenic drug, that it is evil and causes death. Drugs degenerate the body and lead to physical and mental ruin. Quite contrary to the effects of lethal and illegal drugs, Ayahuasca regenerates the human body, strengthens personality development and awakens or matures the human consciousness. Ayahuasca is actually an effective medicine in healing drug dependencies. A successful experience in this regard is the Centro Takiwasi de Tarapoto, which has supplemented academic medicine with traditional medicine and developed an alternative model of professional medical treatment to combat addictions.

When one speaks of a hallucinogen or hallucination, one refers to a pathological state. The hallucination is a cheat; it is an illusion, it is a perception without object, it is to see something that doesn't exist. In contrast, Ayahuasca is a dis-hallucinogenic, because it allows us to perceive reality as it is and to break away from the cultural and social hallucination that we are trapped within. Ayahuasca breaks this illusion, alienation or disposition. It awakens and presents the world and life how they are. The best way to put your feet on the ground is to drink Ayahuasca and awaken from all of our sociocultural hallucinations. In the Ayahuasca trance, one sees things that exist in other dimensions or in other realities because there is not just one reality, rather, there are various realities that form an integral reality.

When the first conquering priests entered the Amazon jungle, they described Ayahuasca ceremonies as idolatry or satanic practices. Because of this vilification and demonization, Ayahuasca was related to something demonic. However, the experience of drinking Ayahuasca is to confront the most profound fears, dreads, and anxieties. The trance is a confrontation with our own "demons" or psychic phantasms; it is a passage through our own hell, to arrive at a profound catharsis, to ascend to the heavens, that is, to arrive at balance, health and harmony. Among other infamies, they say that Ayahuasca creates madness and death. This statement is misleading because what Ayahuasca produces is a mystical experience of a symbolic death, which is experienced as if this death was real and the person is reborn, discarding all that was negative in his life and beginning a new life. The significance of this experience of rebirth through a symbolic death is the development of the personality and the consolidation of a new consciousness.

And with respect to madness, we understand that one way of developing our consciousness is to put into question all of our assumptions or self-evident truths. Put precisely, Ayahuasca subjects us to more intense analysis and the questioning of all our presumptions, upon which we base our existence. Many of our ideas about life may be wrong, and these mistakes in the way we understand life and "reality" can lead us to errors, creating physical and mental abnormalities or diseases within us.

The Ayahuasca trance specifically allows us to put into question all "truths" so that they can be clarified or reaffirmed with new and richer perspectives of understanding. The Ayahuasca trance, in that moment, can create a crisis of our limited understanding. Faced with this crisis, human weakness does not want to recognize the new perspectives of understanding that are revealed. This is a reactionary attitude that, faced with the crisis of our thoughts, causes the panic of madness to arise.

In essence, Ayahuasca is a serious matter that one should enter into well informed. Ayahuasca is a very special medicine and the personal mysticism that can be developed requires a combination of commitment and discipline. Finally, the true positive results of physical wellness and personal development that can be achieved with Ayahuasca debunks all of the disinformation and reaffirms it as a sacred medicine, the Mother of all mothers.

Ronald Rivera Cachique is an Ayahuasquero and owner of the shamanic centerAyahuasca Sabiduria. He is be featured prominently in the documentary "The Path of the Sun," born on October 27, 1967, in the city of Pucallpa, the capital of the Amazon region of Ucayali in Peru. He studied philosophy in the Human Sciences program at La Universidad Nacional Mayor de San Marco a State University in Lima Peru. He is also one of the traditional Shamans who works with the "Instituto Nimairama" a transcultural institution dedicated to integrating healthcare, sacred plant medicine and the knowledge and wisdom of native and indigenous shamanism.

AYAHUASCA PROGRAM

Ronald Rivera Cachique's program for a one week treatment with Ayahuasca was the following scheme:

Instructions
- Diet – starts one day before taking the Ayahuasca. The diet is important and its aim to minimize the experience of being stimulated by food, so all the attention can go to the process of healing. No candy, no meat, no spices, no interesting food, a minimum of salt. The breakfast was fruit at 8AM and lunch at 11AM was plain white rice with boiled beans or lentils and a simple salad. Thereafter only water, and after 3PM nothing more.
- No drugs, no alcohol, no sex.
- During the day we stay silent, doing nothing, just resting. "Relax," said Ronald.

Plan for the 11-day-retreat
- Day 1: Tobacco ceremony. Tea made from tobacco leaves was ingested followed by four litres of lukewarm water (40 degrees Celsius), which was given to make the participant puke.
- Day 2-6: Ayahuasca every day – Wednesday could be skipped if too much was happening and/or the dose thursday could be smaller.
- Day 7-11: Do nothing, stay with the process of healing.

Site for the retreat

Nature, if possible jungle.

THE AYAHUASCA DIARIES

Every day we keep a diary describing the event of the night before. Here extracts for the diary by the first author:

May 20, 2014: Tobacco ceremony. I feared this one, knowing that tobacco tea is poisonous, so I would most likely die, if I did not manage to puke. I really did not like the idea! I was very surprised over the strong therapeutic effect of the ritual. I vomited four times– each time about a litre of water and tobacco tea. Every time I went deeper down into my body, as if layers of old dirt were removed. I did not manage to vomit all the way down from my pelvis during the ritual, but at 3 AM I had to get out of bed to puke again, and this time I did…

May 21, 2014: First Ayahuasca session. I took the 40ml of Ayahuasca (containing estimated 20-40 mg of DMT) Ronald measured up for me in a measure-glass; the tea was brown, thick and creamy like chocolate with a somewhat pleasant taste of wood, herbs and soil. Not much happened to begin with. We were meditating for an hour, just sitting and watching. Ronald was sitting still like a statue, without a movement at all during this hour – except for a few big, actually enormous, cigarettes. I was kind of disappointed, expecting a stronger hallucinogenic effect. Then I decided to have a more active attitude and I asked Ayahuasca to teach me what it had to teach. At the same time Ronald started to sing very beautifully; it was very deep songs…

> The sacred medicine Ayahuasca
> Knows how to heal us, knows how to treat us,
> The sacred medicine Ayahuasca
> It cures you, it cures me, it cures us
> The sacred medicine Ayahuasca
> It heals us, it elevates us.

Slowly, very slowly, and very sweetly, it started to take me into the world of energy and vibrations. The sound of the jungle, normally quite low, raised into a gigantic noise, metallic and horrible. I was not this, this was insects and birds from the jungle, I was something else…

Little by little the Ayahuasca tea showed me that this I am also. Then it came to my body, and it was like one curled line after the other straightened out. Very gently, very slowly, very sweetly. I was not brutal like LSD or magical mushrooms (psilocybin); it was healing me on a much deeper level than the mescaline containing cactus.

Ayahuasca showed me all the small physical moves my spine and pelvis had not done for years. I confronted all my adult and well-conditioned stiffness. Little by little I started to feel a physical strength I had not felt for years. It continued to build up for a long time. In the end I felt like a strong ape, or like a panther, a mighty predator. It was amazing. I had a body like a panther, but I was 1,000 times more intelligent than a panther. What a wonder the human being is!

I was in a good mood, and the universe of life continued to open up. Ayahuasca went systematically through my body, and cured my bad left shoulder, my balls and other places that badly needed cure and attention. I understood that Ayahuasca was medicine, and said "Buene medicina" to Ronald, who laughed.

Pavlina was in trouble; she asked me to come over and help her, so I asked Ronald if I could go to her, and he said yes. I did, and she was confused about what was happening now and what was happening in the past. I helped her as well as I could, and song for her, a song I made for her in the moment, happy and silly. She laughed like a baby.

I went back to my own place and Ayahuasca took me deeper. I felt that the dose was too small, a thought I had from the very beginning… Obviously Pavlina had the opposite experience. It was way too much for her, she said.

May 22, 2014: Second Ayahuasca session. I asked for more Ayahuasca than Ronald wanted to give me, but he gave me 60 ml instead of the normal 40ml, when he measured it up. In spite of that nothing happened for hours. Absolutely nothing unusual happened. I got more and more frustrated, tired and disappointed, and at the time I judged to be the time for the peak of the trip I bought in to the thought that "Maybe Ayahuasca does not work on me." In the end I had to share my frustration with Ronald, so I said: "I am tired, I want to go to sleep. Nothing is happening, absolutely nothing!" Ronald came to me, and said quietly:

"Tranquille. Tomorrow a different type of Ayahuasca." "Oh", I thought, "so he has used a weaker type of Ayahuasca today. That explains it." Later I learned that this was not the case.

But this made me relax, and I laid down; about 10 seconds after I felt the inner clue of the hallucinogen, and then about a minute later it opened up totally and took me away. I was again in the world of magical life, made of patterned energy full of meaning. But something was not right.

"Vomit?" said Ronald, and that seemed like a good idea, so I started to vomit, not my stomach content as usually, but all the alien energies I have accumulated through my life – other peoples energies I have taken in. The purification continued for a long time, it felt like hours. Ronald sang a song about vomiting, and other very good, kind, happy, playful, and friendly Ayahuasca songs, and that helped a lot.

And then I was again the panther, the totally strong and healthy body, fast as lightening, and free to move in a thousand ways. Wow, so much strength and power in this beautiful, awesome body.

Now my trip had finally started, and it really took off! But Ronald wanted to go to bed, and end the session. I accepted it, as I felt fine. But I was not really fine. I could not walk. Pavlina had to support me to the bed, where I managed to take the mosquito net down, before I felt to sleep a few minutes later. I woke up, relaxed, happy, a bit wasted, with a mosquito bite on my hand.

May 23, 2014: Third Ayahuasca session. Again I got the normal dose of Ayahuasca plus a little – about 60 ml. The swallowing was not pleasant today, I felt nausea right away. The effect came fast, but not very intense to start with.

But I knew that I had gone deeper, and this day Ayahuasca started to work on my anus, where I for a long time have had some problems of unknown causes. I did not consider the problems big enough to seek help. Ayahuasca spoke to me: "You must take this seriously. It is a tumour. It can kill you." And there was certainly a tumour there, of the size 2x2x2 cm or so, in the left side of my anus. Then Ayahuasca shoved me a picture I have had for a long time of my asshole: brown and curled and ugly – so much shame and disgust there!

I didn´t realize for my whole life that this was how I really felt about my ass - and about my genitals also for that sake! Horrible. I followed the shame and disgust back to its origin and met again mother, this time in a totally crazy and dysfunctional version. A mother trained as a nurse, who truly hated "bacteria," the ultimate enemy of man - and with that all kind of bodily excretions.

I was for some reason not concerned with Ayahuasca diagnoses, which translated to medical language meant "Carcinoma in situ, possibly anal cancer," but I understood that this session was very timely, and that I had to surrender totally to Ayahuasca's healing and cure. This was simply my chance to heal! I needed purification and healing so much more than I thought!

I lay down and allowed the medicine to work; Ayahuasca took me again to the world of biological information, but this time I did not feel strong like a panther; I felt depressed, and I realized that this depression had been with me for many years. I had denied it. I had pretended that all was well with me. But it was not: I was not happy, I was depressed. And my body suffered from this depression.

Again Pavlina called for help, but at first I did not feel like going to her; what I worked on was a bit more important than Pavlina! Then I realized that we are in this together and that we in this beautiful relationship help each other out and that Pavlina actually is the one saving and healing me, so I went to her to assist her. I stayed with her for a long time. After an hour or so she let me return to my own madras so I could continue my process.

I felt blessed that Ayahuasca finally had come to cure my ass and my shame. This was the third session of five, and the third healing day of the 10 day retreat, so much could still be healed. But I had to focus, and not allow my attention to get of the problem. I need to continuously ask for the healing - and I need to open myself up to receive it.

Again I could not walk out when Ronald finished the session about 11:30PM, but I had to crawl like a baby. I laughed hard all the way to my bed, and Pavlina supported me like an old lady. "Ayahuasca is good energy" said Ronald and for some reason this was very funny. This day the tumour was photographed (see figure 1).

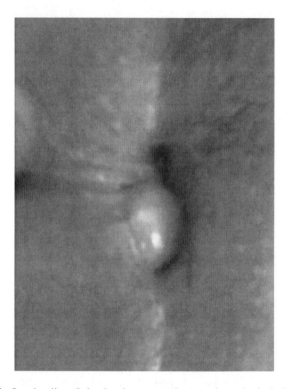

Figure 1. Anal tumour before healing. It is clearly seen and approximately 2x2x2 cm in size.

May 24, 2014: Fourth Ayahuasca session. In the beginning of this session I got a memory of being an embryo. I relived ontogenesis and this was like a celebration of a truly amazing state, where consciousness draws on all the information from billions of years of evolution and of the collected information creating the human form including all the organs and structures of the body. At the same time it was clear that consciousness was not limited to the body. The embryo also followed what happens around it.

I got this feeling that I need to be like an embryo to heal. I needed to go back to this state, where consciousness was one with the body and its surroundings. I needed to go all the way back to live to heal. This time I felt Ayahuasca from the very beginning of the session. It started just after swallowing the brown thick puree that was much less tasty than yesterday.

And yet Ayahuasca didn't open to me. For a very long time I was watching and there was this little silent movement of energy, but nothing happened.

I had this thought that dose was too small and nothing would happen. I laid down in the hope that this would intensify the process. I touched the tumour in my ass and it felt less alien than yesterday, like something good happened to it. The physical contact with the tumour opens up for some feelings. Mostly fear. It was like there was energetic tension between the body and the tumour that needed to be levelled out. So I called Ayahuasca to help heal my body.

I was lying for a long time and not much happened. Then I relaxed and I came back to tumour again and again, maybe ten times. But not much happened. Again I got frustrated and impatient. This continued for long time. It was like I gave up. And suddenly Ayahuasca came from "underneath" - from inside my body - and called upon my consciousness. It put me in, it took me completely. It was as if I was sinking into water, turning into a thick fluid of energy, patterns and life.

The most beautiful world of patterns opened up for me and I realized that as life I am these patterns. My life is these patterns. My consciousness is these patterns. I kept sinking into this. But something was not right. There was a conflict, some bad energy. I touched my ass again. There was a weird double experience to watch my body from outside with my fingers and be this ocean of this energy and information at the same time. I was again touching on the question of my depression.

Ronald asked: Janu are you ok? I couldn't say yes and no wasn't right either. So I said: "maybe!."

Pavlina came to me and tried to support me and Ronald came and blew smoke on my head and spread perfumed water on my body. Do you want song or silence, asked Ronald? Silence, I said.

At this point Ayahuasca got more and more intense. The light in my body lit in more colours then there are in the spectrum of light, and the energy was vibrating and dancing. So much life! Gradually the tension disappears and I was happily one with what is. I still felt, or rather Ayahuasca told me, that there was a deeper level of awakeness and presence and that I have to go there to heal genuinely. The session was over. I was on Ayahuasca more than ever, but very peaceful and ready to go – or more correctly crawl – to sleep.

May 25, 2014: Fifth Ayahuasca session. This session was far the most intense. It was really difficult to swallow the Ayahuasca and the effect was there almost before I drank it. In this session I had to go through a lot of strong, negative emotions.

Pavlina turned the camera off before the Inca song I really wanted to record and that made me to almost explode with anger. I stayed with the anger and Ayahuasca took me back to my early childhood, where my parents were so angry with me always. It was totally meaningless; they were truly crazy. I touched my tumour in my ass again, and I felt endless shame. My asshole was the most charged tissue in my body; my parents just hated everything about shit and diapers, and the feeling of their shallow care and disgust of me was horrible.

But then I found a deeper layer yet; my mother desired me sexually and was ashamed over it; endlessly ashamed and that was really the shame I felt. Ayahuasca took me still deeper; I sank into the world of life energy, conscious; a vibrating, pulsating energy in a thousand patterns and colours that gave shape and form and meaning to all life in me and around me. I stared in awe like forever at these patterns; I was consciousness witnessing the life I also am...

Words cannot express what I saw. Again and again Ayahuasca took me back in time, to show me that I was hanging in old stuff that should be let go of.

I felt sadness for all the failures and losses in my life, and I realized that all is well; I need to take the learning, then nothing is lost and nothing has been without a reason. Life is learning, but we need to take the learning. I felt fresh, totally alive, here and now, and past was no more. I touch my tumour again, and strong pulses of negative energy came out of it, like shockwaves; like it was a battery that finally got uncharged. So much shame! I understood why my asshole was my sorest spot; why I was likely to develop a tumour here.

In the end of the session I was happy to feel that the tumour felt like only being half as big as before. When I woke up next morning, it was still smaller. I was definitely healing. But I was sad; some old feelings were still in me and had still to go. I felt still very much on Ayahuasca and I felt confident that the process would continue, and that I, with Pavlina´s help, would get cured. I was definitely healing, on so many levels at the same time!

One month later the anal tumour had disappeared completely as it can be seen on a picture from day 30 (see figure 2).

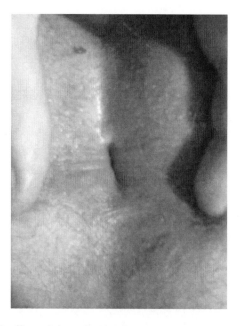

Figure 2. Anal tumour after healing – it is no longer there.

Pavlina´s Ayahuasca diary

May 20, 2014: Tobacco ceremony. I felt happy, this is why I came here and yet I was bit scared of the vomiting part. Dark coloured tea with very strong smell. Taste was bad (especially the tale), but not horrible. My body is one big tension full of expectations and mind is in alert. While we are slowly drinking warm water Ronald started to sing. After the first litre I vomited and after second and third nothing.

I got troubled. I had a lot of thoughts and doubts. Am I ok? Am I doing it right? Why am I not vomiting as much as Søren? Did I puke enough or will I die poisoned by tobacco? Does it mean that I am pure? It cannot be. Maybe I had my share of vomiting last year when I was sick.

I was very grateful for a calm energy of Ronald and his songs. I am leaving the ceremony worried, with a feeling of failure, but the feeling is slowly disappearing and in the end I am happy.

May 21, 2014: First Ayahuasca session. I am a bit nervous, but it is ok. From my experiences with LSD I expect this to be a wonderful experience of healing. Ronald is giving me smoothie like liquid of brown-reddish colour and the taste is not bad at all. At the beginning I am disappointed, not much is happening, some sensations in the body, some visions, no wisdom, no understanding. At one moment I consider myself to be sober and I am ready to finish the session.

Then a kind of inner dialog started. Both voices are mine. One is wise, "the Ayahuasca me" who knows everything and the other is my well known "normal" me. I asked Ayahuasca to free me from slavery of the body. I got the choice: "Do you want to be free or do you want to change and improve your body to be beautiful?"

Now it is time to be honest so I asked back: "Can I have both?" The answer was immediate: "Yes, you can have everything." Sure thing: "Then I want everything." I see a picture that symbolizes all I want. It is a lot. Nothing happened for a while and I thought I prefer LSD more. "You love the body" the voice said and to my surprise I answered: "yes I do, can you show me what is more wonderful then my body?"

Then colourful visions started. Very abstract, geometric with the theme of good night stories for kids and the echo of my name twisted in childish ways, feeling of being a very little girl, happy, full of energy, in the ecstasy, very sexual. Ronald started to sing and suddenly the patterns of my visions became more structural, dimensional and I was looking up at Ronald singing and standing above me and between us there was a weird web of dead lianas. This is important there is some understanding for me, I thought. But then Ronald stopped to sing and suddenly I got lost in the incredible noise of the jungle, colours, everything was shaking, fragments of visions and sensations in my body. It was overwhelming. I am confused and thoughts sprang out of me: This is too much. I cannot stand this. I need peace. Please stop. Make it go away. I want this to be over. I have a bad trip. I will never ever do that again! I want to go home. I am opened my eyes to have a peace from visions, but everything is shaking and noise seemed louder so I'm closed them again. "

I need help. Ronald is asking me if I am ok and I said no. He is talking to me, but I don't understand and I feel like I need to understand this mess. It doesn't make any sense. I need Søren. I'm calling and he is coming. "Ask for teaching," he said "Ayahuasca is teaching you." "You wanted everything and this is it, this is the life."

I need him to speak and yet the words makes sense just for a very short moment and then I am again overwhelmed. Slowly it starts to sink in. "This is not true, this is old, these are thoughts I believed in, this is not too much, this is life. That was then, when you were little; this is your mother's position and not yours."

With the combination of Søren's talk and Ronald's song I am coming out of confusion to celebrate life, back to ecstasy, incredible sweetness. I am the sweetest flower of the world. I feel like a little girl again. Everything is sweet. To be alive is so sweet. I am. I love my mom; I understand how difficult it was for her. I love her. I am very grateful to Ronald and Søren.

May 22, 2014: Second Ayahuasca session. I feel nervous. In an attempt to avoid the last night crises I have been praying all day to Ayahuasca for teaching. Ronald asked us if we want a smaller dose, I say normal but I am worried if this is good idea. I sat calmly for an hour, waiting for effect to come. I felt sick in the stomach and I had diarrhoea. "Purification" I thought. I felt Ayahuasca started to work and I prayed to ease the panic that took me. For while there are unpleasant feelings and visions, but then I opened and the teaching started: "You don't need anybody. You are not small. You don't need help. All is well. You are fine. It was just an illusion that you are small and weak. You can let go of it."

My attention is flowing to different part of my body. The healing of the body started. "You don't have to turn yourself into your mother's body-shape, you are fine." I see how I made myself ugly to support my mother out of love and how this change love in to sourness, ugliness and anger. "You don't have to make yourself ugly to please your mother." "I see all the women in my family and how they did the same and how the sourness carved their body." The healing of the body again. We are healing my family. I love you, mom.

I think. LSD is the father and Ayahuasca is the mother. Such a good mother, loving and caring. "All men are the father and all women are the mother. You are safe. All is well, Child of the Universe. You are safe and loved."

Healing of the body. Søren is troubled, nothing is happening for him. I said a few words to him and dive in to the love. I love him, I want to help him, and I want to show my love. "Love is. You don't have to do anything. You don't have to show it, it doesn't have to be expressed any way. Love just is. There is just love. Surrender to love."

Healing of the body. Søren vomited. I feel this is good. I have this thought and sentence for him: "You are not empty, you are full. Surrender to the love. You don't have to help or do anything for anybody. You don't have to please anybody. Søren is well, better he will find out himself, and then you interfere. Love just is. Surrender to love."

Healing of the body. "I love him. But if there is just love, there is no me. Who am I, who is Søren?" "There is nobody and nothing. Only emptiness. "

May 23, 2014: Third Ayahuasca session. I was a little nervous, but not much at all. Last night was so wonderful and happy, so all is well. Thanks to diet my senses are sharper and that causes the drink to be really discusting. One hour of waiting and silence is fine, I feel good. Then I saw a big tick on my belly and I understood that this night will be about fear. I saw big machines with drills and robots. " You are like a robot." Ayahuasca said to me.

Suddenly there were a lot of pictures about how fear is used during the raising of a child to control, restrict, to create obedience to authorities. "You are not alive; you are a robot." That made me sad. I understood. Fear is not real; it is made to give power to authorities. This is just an illusion I repeat to myself and hope that I will reach the happy state. Where is my happiness, it is my right to be happy. I'm falling into a dark hole. Full of thoughts: This is sad. This night is bad. This is leading nowhere. It is so dark. I'm weak. I'm tired. I want out. There is no way out. I'm confused. Ronald's songs are annoying today. I had diarrhoea again and I could hardly control my body.

I talk with Søren; he was helping me from his position. He says I'm fine, but when it is so dark and visions full of metallic sounds and pictures of death, body is shaking, I don't feel fine. Eventually he is coming to me. "You are an embryo," he said. That makes sense. I feel conflict of me coming and my mother's position "Don't come, only if I can have my first daughter also. Don't come if I cannot have her." I feel stuck. What to do? I'm coming anyway. "This is fucked up." Søren's voice makes me calmer. Thinks are getting better, but in the silence it gets bad again. I'm afraid to close my eyes, but I'm so tired.

This is horror. I don't want this anymore. "You are healing," said Søren. "Ok," I said. But I don't like this healing. "Trust the life," Ayahuasca said to me. Eventually and very slowly I became better. When Ronald sang happy Inca songs we were singing with him. "Wow! I thought that things are permanent. But this is not true." I felt much better but still with a bitter feeling of failure. I'm not free yet, I didn't get it. We went to sleep, but my process continues. I still had a fear of falling asleep and I repeated to myself mantra: Trust the life, trust the life….

Next day I still felt Ayahuasca in the body and Søren said that this is good, I'm healing. I was clinging to that all day.

May 24, 2014: Fourth Ayahuasca session. I asked Ronald for a smaller dose since I was feeling Ayahuasca in the body all day. I sit peacefully and keeping in the mind our talk with Søren from this morning – The patterns and weird visions are the energy and how everything is made. To heal I need to see it and feel it and Ayahuasca is showing me what I don't know about myself and the world. Healing is when I become conscious.

The teaching started. I saw how the Universe is made and its complexity. My body is vibrating. Then I see how I'm using the feelings like a guidance or path I follow blindly. I believe that feelings are ultimate truth. Like this feeling I'm cold – immediately I go for blanket in my blindness. I look again on the energy to try to understand what is happening. Then I see it – my body full of movement, patterns, complex and active is meeting cold air. Cold air has different patterns emptier, slow and I perceive it as a cold. Meeting is influencing the body and activity in it is slowing down. It brings the change and I hate changes. I want things to be as they are, as I know them, so I know how to behave and what to do. Makes me feel safe.

Wow I didn't know. I hate changes. It is miracle that I'm actually here whit this attitude. Then Ayahuasca is showing me how the healing works. How the consciousness creates patterns of matter, atoms, molecules, and cells. And this is how everything is made. Sickness is a disturbance on the level of consciousness. Feelings and thoughts are creating their own patterns that disturb the harmony of consciousness. To heal you have to allow consciousness to flow naturally. Everything is consciousness.

Then I see all kind of disturbance in the body and I'm healing. In the end I see weird energy on the spine under the neck, but I don't understand it yet. But it is ok, it will come. Energy is shifting and I felt that Søren needed support. Ronald feels that too and asked him if everything is ok. Søren referred that not much is happening. I gave all my blankets to him and eventually I sat next to him and love him and support him. My session is over.

May 25, 2014: Fifth Ayahuasca session. This is the final teaching. Nothing else is more important than this. Experiences, visions or thoughts are not important at all.

> Things are simple.
> Things are as they are.
> Everything is perfect.
> It is our birth-right to be happy.
> It is our natural state to be happy.
> I AM

Discussion

Ayahuasqueros regard both mental and physical diseases to be essentially psychosomatic. The cause of disease is always something unconscious, something oppressed. What is oppressed and held by our unconscious is the life events from which a strong negative (or positive) emotional charge that is unbearable for us in the moment. The oppression works by sending the negative energy into our body to be kept there for later integration and learning. The oppressed energies are causing disease and compromised functioning of body and mind. The loss of consciousness in the disease process is reversed by the enlightening given by the Ayahuasca ceremony.

It is very important to understand that it is NOT the Ayahuasca tea in itself that heals, but the ceremony where the shaman supports the traveller in meeting himself and his oppressed material. The philosophy of the Ayahuasqueros is therefore of essential importance for the process of healing.

The healing follows the simple scheme: Feel, understand and let go of your negative beliefs. It is thus not different from the process of healing in holistic medicine in general. We refer to our six new textbooks on evidence-based holistic mind-body medicine for further reading on this (44-49).

This study has all the weaknesses of a qualitative and theoretical approach. Systematic clinical trials of Ayahuasca or similar hallucinogenic substances like LSD, psilocybin or mescaline should be done with a series of patients having the major physical and mental disorders to truly establish the curative effects of the Ayahuasca.

Ayahuasca have been used for thousands of years in South and Central America. It is known to have no serious side effects, and it seems to be a very effective medicine; there exist a few reports of suspected severe adverse effects, but these have not been seen systematically and could be caused by other things than Ayahuasca (50-61).

The strategy for its use and the philosophy kept by the Ayahuasqueros seems to be of essential importance for the effect of the healing ritual (62-67). The hallucinogenic drug seems to be of less importance than the philosophy and practical setting of the ritual. The hallucinogenic effect seems to speed the natural process of healing and learning up, so it can be done in days instead of taking a life time. There seems to be no major difference in the hallucinogenic effect of Ayahuasca and LSD. It seems rational to use LSD-25 in clinical research with hallucinogens as medicine as the dose and time of the trip are difficult to control when using Ayahuasca. We have estimated the effect of a normal Ayahuasca trip to be equivalent to a middle sized LSD trip. The effect of Ayahuasca lasts for 6-8 hours, which is very similar to LSD.

DMT itself has a much shorter effect, so in clinical trials we recommend use of the original potion Ayahuasca, or LSD as a substitute for this. The problem is that every Ayahuasquero has his own recipe; according to shamans we talked with there are some potions even without DMT. We do not consider these types of Ayahuasca effective, as we see the DMT as the active component. A variety of trips with unknown content are sold to frustrated tourists at a high price by colourful "modern shamans." It is therefore of high importance to engage with competent shamans who work in the original tradition of the Amazonian Ayahuasqueros.

CONCLUSION

It seems clear that Ayahuasca and the other strong hallucinogens work in the same way and have the same mind-expanding effect. This effect can be used as medicine for a long range of mental and physical diseases, like depression or some cancers for example, if used in the right setting, where it is backed up by a sound philosophy of life and a deep understanding of the process of healing.

The Native Americans of the Amazon jungle and the adjacent regions have for thousands of years developed the use of hallucinogens as medicine, and the best Ayahuasqueros today are eminent doctors able to help their patients with many medical problem they come with. There are today unfortunately also many fake shamans that make a living from selling Ayahuasca trips to the many naive tourists that every year visit Peru and South America. To continue the important job to take the traditional knowledge of Shamanistic medicine to the developed world it is of paramount importance to work with serious and qualified Ayahuasqueros.

We found the scheme of Ronald Rivera Cachique to be close to perfect, and recommend this to be the starting point of further research in the use of medical hallucinogens. He emphasized a simple diet, an 11 day retreat with five days of Ayahuasca in a row. The retreat must happen in the nature and the participants must be passive and reflective for 11 days.

Thus the optimal way to use Ayahuasca and the other strong hallucinogens as medicine seems to be a system with five consecutive days of Ayahuasca/hallucinogens, supported by a shaman/Ayahuasquero/spiritual teacher who is trained in philosophy of life, allowing the patient to go deeper into the unconscious every day. The active phase of the treatment is then followed by five days of silent reflection and contemplation. This strategy seems to be the traditional way to use Ayahuasca and an extremely effective scheme for healing both physical and mental disorder. It seems rational to use LSD-25 in clinical research with hallucinogens as medicine as the dose and time of the trip are difficult to control when using Ayahuasca.

ACKNOWLEDGMENTS

The Danish Quality of Life Survey, Quality of Life Research Center and the Research Clinic for Holistic Medicine, Copenhagen, was from 1987 till today supported by grants from the 1991 Pharmacy Foundation, the Goodwill-fonden, the JL-Foundation, E Danielsen and Wife's Foundation, Emmerick Meyer's Trust, the Frimodt-Heineken Foundation, the Hede Nielsen

Family Foundation, Petrus Andersens Fond, Wholesaler CP Frederiksens Study Trust, Else and Mogens Wedell-Wedellsborg's Foundation and IMK Almene Fond. The research in quality of life and scientific complementary and holistic medicine was approved by the Copenhagen Scientific Ethical Committea under the numbers (KF)V. 100.1762-90, (KF)V. 100.2123/91, (KF)V. 01-502/93, (KF)V. 01-026/97, (KF)V. 01-162/97, (KF)V. 01-198/97, and further correspondence. We declare no conflicts of interest.

REFERENCES

[1] Desmarchelier C, Gurni A, Ciccia G, Giulietti AM. Ritual and medicinal plants of the Ese'ejas of the Amazonian rainforest (Madre de Dios, Peru). J Ethnopharmacol 1996;52(1):45-51.
[2] de Rios MD, Grob CS. Ayahuasca use in cross-cultural perspective. J Psychoactive Drugs 2005;37(2):119-21.
[3] Dobkin de Rios M. Ayahuasca--the healing vine. Int J Soc Psychiatry 1971;17(4):256-69.
[4] Dobkin de Rios M. The vidente phenomenon in third world traditional healing: An Amazonian example. Med Anthropol 1984;8(1):60-70.
[5] Andritzky W. Sociopsychotherapeutic functions of ayahuasca healing in Amazonia. J Psychoactive Drugs 1989;21(1):77-89.
[6] Arrevalo G. Interview with Guillermo Arrevalo, a Shipibo urban shaman, by Roger Rumrrill. Interview by Roger Rumrrill. J Psychoactive Drugs 2005;37(2):203-7.
[7] Blainey MG. Forbidden therapies: Santo Daime, Ayahuasca, and the prohibition of entheogens in Western Society. J Relig Health 2014 Jan 30. [Epub ahead of print]
[8] de Araujo DB, Ribeiro S, Cecchi GA, Carvalho FM, Sanchez TA, Pinto JP, et al. Seeing with the eyes shut: Neural basis of enhanced imagery following Ayahuasca ingestion. Hum Brain Mapp 2012;33(11):2550-60.
[9] de Rios MD, Grob CS, Lopez E, da Silviera DX, Alonso LK, Doering-Silveira E. Ayahuasca in adolescence: Qaualitative results. J Psychoactive Drugs 2005;37(2):135-9.
[10] Agurell S, Holmstedt B, Lindgren JE. Alkaloid content of Banisteriopsis rusbyana. Am J Pharm Sci Support Public Health 1968;140(5):148-51.
[11] Bouso JC, F?bregas JM, Antonijoan RM, Rodr?guez-Fornells A, Riba J. Acute effects of ayahuasca on neuropsychological performance: differences in executive function between experienced and occasional users. Psychopharmacology (Berl) 2013;230(3):415-24.
[12] Bullis RK. The "vine of the soul" vs. the Controlled Substances Act: implications of the hoasca case. J Psychoactive Drugs 2008;40(2):193-9.
[13] Callaway JC. Fast and slow metabolizers of Hoasca. J Psychoactive Drugs 2005;37(2):157-61.
[14] Callaway JC. Various alkaloid profiles in decoctions of Banisteriopsis caapi. J Psychoactive Drugs 2005;37(2):151-5.
[15] Callaway JC, Brito GS, Neves ES. Phytochemical analyses of Banisteriopsis caapi and Psychotria viridis. J Psychoactive Drugs 2005;37(2):145-50.
[16] Callaway JC, Raymon LP, Hearn WL, McKenna DJ, Grob CS, Brito GS, et al. Quantitation of N,N-dimethyltryptamine and harmala alkaloids in human plasma after oral dosing with ayahuasca. J Anal Toxicol 1996;20(6):492-7.
[17] de Rios MD, Grob CS, Baker JR. Hallucinogens and redemption. J Psychoactive Drugs 2002;34(3):239-48.
[18] Deuloufeu V. Chemical constituents isolated from Banisteriopsis and related species. Psychopharmacol Bull 1967;4(3):17-8.
[19] Doering-Silveira E, Grob CS, de Rios MD, Lopez E, Alonso LK, Tacla C, et al. Report on psychoactive drug use among adolescents using ayahuasca within a religious context. J Psychoactive Drugs 2005;37(2):141-4.

[20] Dos Santos RG, Grasa E, Valle M, Ballester MR, Bouso JC, Nomdedeu JF, Homs R, Barbanoj MJ, Riba J. Pharmacology of ayahuasca administered in two repeated doses. Psychopharmacology (Berl) 2012;219(4):1039-53.
[21] Frecska E, More CE, Vargha A, Luna LE. Enhancement of creative expression and entoptic phenomena as after-effects of repeated ayahuasca ceremonies. J Psychoactive Drugs 2012;44(3): 191-9.
[22] Gambelunghe C, Aroni K, Rossi R, Moretti L, Bacci M. Identification of N,N-dimethyltryptamine and beta-carbolines in psychotropic ayahuasca beverage. Biomed Chromatogr 2008;22(10):1056-9.
[23] Grob CS, McKenna DJ, Callaway JC, Brito GS, Neves ES, Oberlaender G, et al. Human psychopharmacology of hoasca, a plant hallucinogen used in ritual context in Brazil. J Nerv Ment Dis 1996;184(2):86-94.
[24] Halpern JH, Sherwood AR, Passie T, Blackwell KC, Ruttenber AJ. Evidence of health and safety in American members of a religion who use a hallucinogenic sacrament. Med Sci Monit 2008;14(8):SR15-22.
[25] Herraiz T, Gonzalez D, Ancin-Azpilicueta C, Aran VJ, Guillen H. Beta-carboline alkaloids in Peganum harmala and inhibition of human monoamine oxidase (MAO). Food Chem Toxicol 2010;48(3):839-45.
[26] Kjellgren A, Eriksson A, Norlander T. Experiences of encounters with ayahuasca--"the vine of the soul." J Psychoactive Drugs 2009;41(4):309-15.
[27] Freedland CS, Mansbach RS. Behavioral profile of constituents in ayahuasca, an Amazonian psychoactive plant mixture. Drug Alcohol Depend 1999;54(3):183-94.
[28] Harris R, Gurel L. A study of ayahuasca use in North America. J Psychoactive Drugs 2012;44(3):209-15.
[29] Labate BC, Cavnar C. The expansion of the field of research on ayahuasca: Some reflections about the ayahuasca track at the 2010 MAPS "Psychedelic Science in the 21st Century" conference. Int J Drug Policy 2011;22(2):174-8.
[30] Liester MB, Prickett JI. Hypotheses regarding the mechanisms of ayahuasca in the treatment of addictions. J Psychoactive Drugs 2012;44(3):200-8.
[31] Loizaga-Velder A, Verres R. Therapeutic effects of ritual ayahuasca use in the treatment of substance dependence--qualitative results. J Psychoactive Drugs 2014;46(1):63-72.
[32] Luna LE. The healing practices of a Peruvian shaman. J Ethnopharmacol 1984;11(2):123-33.
[33] Marderosian AH, Pinkley HV, Dobbins MF. Native use and occurence of N,N-Dimethyltryptamine in the leaves of Banisteriopsis rusbyana. Am J Pharm Sci Support Public Health 1968;140(5):137-47.
[34] McKenna DJ. Clinical investigations of the therapeutic potential of ayahuasca: rationale and regulatory challenges. Pharmacol Ther 2004;102(2):111-29.
[35] Ott J. Pharmepena-Psychonautics: Human intranasal, sublingual and oral pharmacology of 5-methoxy-N,N-dimethyl-tryptamine. J Psychoactive Drugs 2001;33(4):403-7.
[36] Pinkley HV. Plant admixtures to Ayahuasca, the South American hallucinogenic drink. Lloydia 1969;32(3):305-14.
[37] Riba J, McIlhenny EH, Valle M, Bouso JC, Barker SA. Metabolism and disposition of N,N-dimethyltryptamine and harmala alkaloids after oral administration of ayahuasca. Drug Test Anal 2012;4(7-8):610-6.
[38] Riba J, Barbanoj MJ. Bringing ayahuasca to the clinical research laboratory. J Psychoactive Drugs 2005;37(2):219-30.
[39] Riba J, Valle M, Urbano G, Yritia M, Morte A, Barbanoj MJ. Human pharmacology of ayahuasca: subjective and cardiovascular effects, monoamine metabolite excretion, and pharmacokinetics. J Pharmacol Exp Ther 2003;306(1):73-83.
[40] Santos RG, Landeira-Fernandez J, Strassman RJ, Motta V, Cruz AP. Effects of ayahuasca on psychometric measures of anxiety, panic-like and hopelessness in Santo Daime members. J Ethnopharmacol 2007;112(3):507-13.
[41] Sarris J, McIntyre E, Camfield DA. Plant-based medicines for anxiety disorders, part 2: a review of clinical studies with supporting preclinical evidence. CNS Drugs 2013;27(4):301-19. Erratum in: CNS Drugs 2013;27(8):675.

[42] Schwarz MJ, Houghton PJ, Rose S, Jenner P, Lees AD. Activities of extract and constituents of Banisteriopsis caapi relevant to parkinsonism. Pharmacol Biochem Behav 2003;75(3):627-33.
[43] Thomas G, Lucas P, Capler NR, Tupper KW, Martin G. Ayahuasca-assisted therapy for addiction: results from a preliminary observational study in Canada. Curr Drug Abuse Rev 2013;6(1):30-42.
[44] Ventegodt S, Merrick J. Textbook on evidence-based holistic mind-body medicine: Basic principles of healing in traditional Hippocratic medicine. Book I. New York: Nova Science, 2012.
[45] Ventegodt S, Merrick J. Textbook on evidence-based holistic mind-body medicine: Basic philosophy and ethics of traditional Hippocratic medicine. Book II. New York: Nova Science, 2012.
[46] Ventegodt S, Merrick J. Textbook on evidence-based holistic mind-body medicine: Research, philosophy, economy and politics of traditional Hippocratic medicine. Book VI. New York: Nova Science, 2012.
[47] Ventegodt S, Merrick J. Textbook on evidence-based holistic mind-body medicine: Sexology and traditional Hippocratic medicine. Book V. New York: Nova Science, 2013.
[48] Ventegodt S, Merrick J. Textbook on evidence-based holistic mind-body medicine: Holistic practice of traditional Hippocratic medicine. Book III. New York: Nova Science, 2013.
[49] Ventegodt S, Merrick J. Textbook on evidence-based holistic mind-body medicine: Healing the mind in traditional Hippocratic medicine. Book IV. New York: Nova Science, 2013.
[50] Anderson BT, Labate BC, Meyer M, Tupper KW, Barbosa PC, Grob CS, et al. Statement on ayahuasca. Int J Drug Policy 2012;23(3):173-5.
[51] Barbosa PC, Mizumoto S, Bogenschutz MP, Strassman RJ. Health status of ayahuasca users. Drug Test Anal 2012;4(7-8):601-9.
[52] Barbosa PC, Cazorla IM, Giglio JS, Strassman R. A six-month prospectiveevaluation of personality traits, psychiatric symptoms and quality of life inayahuasca-na?ve subjects. J Psychoactive Drugs 2009;41(3):205-12.
[53] Barbosa PC, Giglio JS, Dalgalarrondo P. Altered states of consciousness and short-term psychological after-effects induced by the first time ritual use of ayahuasca in an urban context in Brazil. J Psychoactive Drugs 2005;37(2):193-201.
[54] Callaway JC, McKenna DJ, Grob CS, Brito GS, Raymon LP, Poland RE, et al. Pharmacokinetics of Hoasca alkaloids in healthy humans. J Ethnopharmacol 1999;65(3):243-56.
[55] dos Santos RG. Safety and side effects of ayahuasca in humans: An overview focusing on developmental toxicology. J Psychoactive Drugs 2013;45(1):68-78.
[56] dos Santos RG. A critical evaluation of reports associating ayahuasca with life-threatening adverse reactions. J Psychoactive Drugs 2013;45(2):179-88.
[57] Labate BC. Consumption of ayahuasca by children and pregnant women: medical controversies and religious perspectives. J Psychoactive Drugs 2011;43(1):27-35.
[58] Riba J, Rodriguez-Fornells A, Urbano G, Morte A, Antonijoan R, Montero M, et al. Subjective effects and tolerability of the South American psychoactive beverage Ayahuasca in healthy volunteers. Psychopharmacology (Berl) 2001;154(1):85-95.
[59] Rios O. [Preliminary aspects of the pharmaco-psychiatric study of the ayahuasca and its active principle]. An Fac Med Lima 1962;45(1-2):22-66. [Spanish]
[60] Rodd R. Reassessing the cultural and psychopharmacological significance of Banisteriopsis caapi: preparation, classification and use among the Piaroa of Southern Venezuela. J Psychoactive Drugs 2008;40(3):301-7.
[61] Samoylenko V, Rahman MM, Tekwani BL, Tripathi LM, Wang YH, Khan SI, et al. Banisteriopsis caapi, a unique combination of MAO inhibitory and antioxidative constituents for the activities relevant to neurodegenerative disorders and Parkinson's disease. J Ethnopharmacol 2010;127(2):357-67.
[62] McKenna DJ. Ayahuasca and human destiny. J Psychoactive Drugs 2005;37(2):231-4.
[63] Naranjo P. Hallucinogenic plant use and related indigenous belief systems in the Ecuadorian Amazon. J Ethnopharmacol 1979;1(2):121-45.
[64] Pages Larraya F. [The meaning of the use of ayahuasca among the Chama(Ese'ejja) natives of Eastern Bolivia: a transcultural study]. Acta Psiquiatr Psicol Am Lat 1979;25(4):253-67. [Spanish]

[65] Trichter S, Klimo J, Krippner S. Changes in spirituality among ayahuasca ceremony novice participants. J Psychoactive Drugs 2009;41(2):121-34.
[66] Tupper KW. The globalization of ayahuasca: harm reduction or benefit maximization? Int J Drug Policy 2008;19(4):297-303.
[67] Winkelman M. Drug tourism or spiritual healing? Ayahuasca seekers in Amazonia. J Psychoactive Drugs 2005;37(2):209-18.

In: Mental and Holistic Health: Some International Perspectives ISBN: 978-1-63483-589-3
Editors: J. Calles Jr., D. Greydanus and J. Merrick   © 2015 Nova Science Publishers, Inc.

Chapter 12

SOUTH AFRICA AND BOTSWANA: TRADITIONAL HEALING AND RITUALIZED CANNIBALISM

Søren Ventegodt, MD, MMedSci, EU-MSc-CAM[1,2,3,4,*] *and Pavlina Kordova*[1,2,3]

[1]Quality of Life Research Center, Copenhagen, Denmark
[2]Research Clinic for Holistic Medicine, Copenhagen, Denmark
[3]Nordic School of Holistic Medicine, Copenhagen, Denmark
[4]Scandinavian Foundation for Holistic Medicine, Sandvika, Norway

ABSTRACT

In Africa many people believe that there is healing properties associated with the organs of the body. Animal organs have some healing power, but human organs are the most powerful for healing humans and of the organs the genitals are considered the most powerful for healing. The younger the person is, the more powerful the healing power of the organ and the organ is most powerful for healing, if it is removed alive and the more painful the removal is, the more powerful medicine can be made from the organs. This African tradition, which can also be found in other societies throughout history, goes against modern concepts of ethics and the Traditional Healers Organization have started a movement to explain away with these myths. We have recently travelled in South Africa and participated in meetings about these issues and relay our experience in this paper.

INTRODUCTION

In May 2015 we traveled to South Africa and Botswana to study traditional healing, invited by the Traditional Healers Organization (THO) and its leader Phepsile Maseko in

---

[*] Correspondence: Søren Ventegodt, MD, MMedSci, EUMSc-CAM, Director, Quality of Life Research Center, Frederiksberg Alle 13A, 2tv, DK-1661 Copenhagen V, Denmark. E-mail: ventegodt@livskvalitet.org

Johannesburg. This organization intents to organize 200,000 traditional healers, primarily Sangomas ("Diviners") from all Africa, but today it is mostly active in South Africa.

The Traditional Healer's Organization invited us to help them solve problems related to ethics. They faced two challenges, one was the government of South Africa wanting to control and restrict them from harmful practices, the other was local disapproval and discontent with the healers in some northern regions of South Africa after a number of killings of primarily children and young people, who were suspected to have been killed by people helping the Sangomas in ritual Muthi (or Muti) killings.

We interviewed central persons in the Traditional Healers Organization to understand what Muthi killings are, and we got the following explanation:

- In Africa many people believe that there is healing properties associated with the organs of the body. Animal organs have some healing power, but human organs are the most powerful for healing humans.
- Of the organs the genitals are considered the most powerful for healing.
- The younger the person is, the more powerful the healing power of the organ.
- The organ is most powerful for healing, if it is removed alive and the more painful the removal is, the more powerful medicin can be made from the organs.

Therefore, when a number of children, mostly girls, where found killed, obviously after torture and mutilation, with their genitals cut away, seemingly while the children were still alive, this left little doubt in the local population that this was the Sangomas harvesting the necessary ingredients for their magical brews.

The superstitions related to Muthi killings have a number of horrible expressions in South Africa, Boswana, and the related countries, i.e. rape of young virgin girls, which is generally believed in many parts of the black population to be able to cure AIDS. This leads to thousands of rapes of children in Africa every year and HIV infection spreading.

The local population has been reacting to the Sangomas, since the systematic and frequent Muthi killings – 14 killings in one region in only one year - which have resulted in media attention in South Africa. In many regions healers have been robbed, lost their houses and property taken over by angry neighbors, they have been beaten, raped and in a number of cases stoned or burned to dead in classical witch-fires. The local violent movements towards the Traditional Healers have not stopped the many Muthi killings in the Northern regions, and the Traditional Healers Organization has reacted strongly by organizing big meetings for the Sangomas on ethics.

MEETING THE SANGOMAS

We were invited to speak to the Sangomas at a meeting of 200 Sangomas in the Limpopo district, where the Muthi killings have been frequent; with mostly women attending the meeting as the female Sangomas often are the victims of violence caused by the hate and fear raised by the medial attention to the Muthi killings.

It turned out during the conference that a major part of income for the Sangomas comes from casting spells. This business works this way that if you have an argument with a neighbor or a rival in business, or somebody you from jealousy or another personal reason would like to weaken or harm, then you can pay a Sangoma to cast a spell on him or her. As soon as he or she learns about the spell it will start impacting, often quite dramatically. This mechanism, called the nocebo effect in medical research, is well known also from other research in Voodo (Vodou, Vodun, Vudu).

The good business of casting spells made the Sangomas quite hostile to the idea that good things come from doing good, and bad things come from doing evil. It simply seemed difficult for many Sangomas to get the idea that if you do harmful things, this invites harmful things to be done to you. Therefore they insisted on continuing to cast spells, while they were complaining about being treated badly by the local population. Also the concept of good and bad did not sit well with the Sangomas; this seemed to be western concepts with little meaning to the native black population of rural South Africa and Botswana. But then again, this has been a practice for thousands of years in Africa, and so has the Muthi killings. The problems for the Sangomas come with the Western culture, the modernization of Africa, and the media that focus on the negative side of the healer's tradition.

Are the Traditional Healers powerful healers? Yes they are. Because of their standing in the society their words simply means a world of difference. If they say that you will get better, you will get better – this is the placebo effect in its most clear and condensed form. I they say that you will get ill, you will get ill, if you believe in the Sangomas.

It was discussed at the Ethics Conference in Limpopo that it was very important that Sangomas did not prescribe rape of virgins as a cure for AIDS. Many Sangomas obviously shared the idea that rape will cure HIV, but THO is doing an important job in informing its members and thus stopping the most superstitious Sangomas from directly recommending rape of virgin girls.

CASE OF MASEGO KGOMO

Masego Kgomo was a 10-year-old South African girl whose body was cut up and her organs sold to a sangoma in Soshanguve, South Africa. The little girl's body was found in bushes near the Mabopane railway station near Pretoria. Brian Mangwale, a 30 year old male, was found guilty of the murder and sentenced to life imprisonment: "The judge said the manner in which she was killed was severely aggravating. There was evidence the girl was still alive when her womb and breast were cut out. They were sold to a traditional healer for R4 800" (1).

HOW CAN WE UNDERSTAND THE SYMBOLISM OF THE TRADITIONAL AFRICAN HEALERS?

If we look that the elements of the Muthi killings that makes the most powerful medicine, it is clear that the symbolism comes from the dualism of the core concepts of life and healing:

- Healthy - sick
- Young - old

- Sexual - asexual
- Dominance and power - dominated, powerless
- Killing, preying - being killed, falling prey
- Eating - being eaten

It is worth a reflection that the Muthi medicine using the human organs is actually a soup boiled on the organs, together with magical herbs and other magical things – very much like the magical witch brew of Disney's cartoon witches.

So Muthi medicine is ritualized cannibalism, and it intends to transfer the health, happiness and sexual power from the victim of the Muthi killing over to you. The myth of Count Dracula from Transylvania who slaughtered countless young girls and women and drank their blood to get their youth, health, strength, beauty and life comes to one's mind. The elements are pretty similar and many forms of power abuse and sexual exploitation rotates around this theme: Transference of what is good, from one to another.

The essence of the Muthi medicine is that the Sangoma transfers life, joy and health from the victim to you, the costumer, motivated partly by the payment you give the Sangoma for his or her service, and partly undoubtedly by the Sangomas own celebration of unlimited power, which is at the core of the Muthi killing rite.

WHAT IS THE FUTURE FOR THE AFRICAN SANGOMAS?

The Traditional Healers Organization (THO) has been strong in distancing itself from all harmful deeds of the Sangomas, like Muthi killings and virgin rapes. The ethical rules of the Sangomas are very clear in forbidding these acts (1). The leaders of THO also believes that the evil deeds are done by "fake Sangomas", nor by the "true Sangomas" who are called to practice and inspired by the divine.

Sangomas have a mighty power in Africa. The WHO has acknowledged them as the doctors of Africa, and there seem to be no alternative to the Sangomas. Yet there is a sharp conflict between the traditional healers practice and a modern and informed Africa that slowly is emerging. The most fundamental problem seems to be that the western concept of good and evil is not shared by the Sangomas or by the people they serve. It seems that many native Africans simply believe in power. In the old Sagas of Iceland we find the statement that "power is right". If you have the power to do a thing, you also have the right to do it. In a modern civilization power and right are two very different things.

The Traditional Healers Organization uses a strange way of communicating the message to its members regarding Muthi killings: You should not be involved in Muthi killings, because this cause troubles to the traditional healers and put the Sangoma's name in a bad light. The argument is not that "you should not torture, molest, rape, and kill children, because it is wrong". We felt that the way THO framed this showed the depth of the problem: You cannot argue with right and wrong, good and bad in Africa, because these concepts are not part of African traditional culture.

We (SV) tried to bring a Christian argument to the ethics conference: "You shall love your neighbor," but this argument had no validity in the assembly as the concept of "love" itself had no meaning to most of the participant Sangomas of the conference.

We were at our arrival sad and surprised to learn that one in three or four women in South Africa has been raped. As we studied the value system behind the Muthi killing and power as the primary value of the black native Africans we understood some of the background for the massive epidemic of rape and violence in South Africa.

THO is a powerful organization which might have the power to teach its members about ethics, good and bad, right and wrong, love versus power, but it will be a long battle of values and only if the South African government sides up with the THO and empowers this organization can we hope for a positive development.

REFERENCES

[1] Life sentence for muti killer. URL: http://www.news24.com/SouthAfrica/News/Life-sentence-for-muti-killer-20111128-4.

[2] Ventegodt S, Molefe M (Dumezweni). Traditional Healers Organization code of ethics 2015. Johannesburg: Traditional Healers Organization, 2015.

SECTION THREE: ACKNOWLEDGMENTS

In: Mental and Holistic Health: Some International Perspectives   ISBN: 978-1-63483-589-3
Editors: J. Calles Jr., D. Greydanus and J. Merrick   © 2015 Nova Science Publishers, Inc.

Chapter 13

ABOUT THE EDITORS

Joseph L Calles Jr., MD, is Associate Professor of Psychiatry, Department of Psychiatry and the Psychiatry Residency Training Program, Western Michigan University Homer Stryker MD School of Medicine, Kalamazoo, Michigan, USA. He is also Clinical Associate Professor of Psychiatry, Michigan State University College of Osteopathic Medicine, East Lansing, Michigan, USA. Dr. Calles received his medical degree from Michigan State University College of Human Medicine, where he also completed his Psychiatry residency. He completed his Child and Adolescent Psychiatry fellowship at Los Angeles County/University of Southern California Medical Center and a member of the American Academy of Child and Adolescent Psychiatry and the National Association for the Dually Diagnosed. Publications and presentations have been in the areas of child and adolescent mood disorders, disruptive behavior disorders, intellectual and developmental disorders, substance use disorders, psychopharmacology, and cults.
    E-mail: joseph.calles@med.wmich.edu

Donald E. Greydanus, MD, Dr. HC (Athens), FAAP, FSAM (Emeritus), FIAP (HON) is Professor and Founding Chair of the Department of Pediatric and Adolescent Medicine, as well as Pediatrics Program Director at the Western Michigan University Homer Stryker MD School of Medicine (WMED), Kalamazoo, Michigan, USA. He is also Professor of Pediatrics and Human Development at Michigan State University College of Human Medicine (East Lansing, Michigan, USA) as well as Clinical Professor of Pediatrics at MSU College of Osteopathic Medicine in East Lansing, Michigan, USA. Received the 1995 American Academy of Pediatrics' Adele D. Hofmann Award for "Distinquished Contributions in Adolescent Health," the 2000 Mayo Clinic Pediatrics Honored Alumnus Award for "National Contributions to the field of Pediatrics," and the 2003 William B Weil, Jr., MD Endowed Distinguished Pediatric Faculty Award from Michigan State University College of Medicine for "National and international recognition as well as exemplary scholarship in pediatrics." Received the 2004 Charles R Drew School of Medicine (Los Angeles, CA) Stellar Award for contributions to pediatric resident education and awarded an honorary membership in the Indian Academy of Pediatrics—an honor granted to only a few pediatricians outside of India. Was the 2007-2010 Visiting Professor of Pediatrics at Athens University, Athens, Greece and received the Michigan State University College of Human Medicine Outstanding Community Faculty Award in 2008. In 2010 he received the title of Doctor Honoris Causa from the

University of Athens (Greece) as a "distinguished scientist who through outstanding work has bestowed praise and credit on the field of adolescent medicine (Ephebiatrics)." In 2010 he received the Outstanding Achievement in Adolescent Medicine Award from the Society for Adolescent Medicine "as a leading force in the field of adolescent medicine and health." In 2014 he was selected by the American Medical Association as AMA nominee for the ACGME Pediatrics Residency Review Committee (RRC) in Chicago, Illinois, USA. Past Chair of the National Conference and Exhibition Planning Group (Committee on Scientific Meetings) of the American Academy of Pediatrics and member of the Pediatric Academic Societies' (SPR/PAS) Planning Committee (1998 to Present). In 2011 elected to The Alpha Omega Alpha Honor Society (Faculty member) at Michigan State University College of Human Medicine, East Lansing, Michigan. Former member of the Appeals Committee for the Pediatrics' Residency Review Committee (RRC) of the Accreditation Council for Graduate Medical Education (Chicago, IL) in both adolescent medicine and general pediatrics. Numerous publications in adolescent health and lectureships in many countries on adolescent health.

E-mail: donald.greydanus@med.wmich.edu

Joav Merrick, MD, MMedSci, DMSc, born and educated in Denmark is professor of pediatrics, child health and human development, Division of Pediatrics, Hadassah Hebrew University Medical Center, Mt Scopus Campus, Jerusalem, Israel and Kentucky Children's Hospital, University of Kentucky, Lexington, Kentucky United States and professor of public health at the Center for Healthy Development, School of Public Health, Georgia State University, Atlanta, United States, the medical director of the Health Services, Division for Intellectual and Developmental Disabilities, Ministry of Social Affairs and Social Services, Jerusalem, the founder and director of the National Institute of Child Health and Human Development in Israel. Numerous publications in the field of pediatrics, child health and human development, rehabilitation, intellectual disability, disability, health, welfare, abuse, advocacy, quality of life and prevention. Received the Peter Sabroe Child Award for outstanding work on behalf of Danish Children in 1985 and the International LEGO-Prize ("The Children's Nobel Prize") for an extraordinary contribution towards improvement in child welfare and well-being in 1987.

E-mail: jmerrick@zahav.net.il

In: Mental and Holistic Health: Some International Perspectives   ISBN: 978-1-63483-589-3
Editors: J. Calles Jr., D. Greydanus and J. Merrick   © 2015 Nova Science Publishers, Inc.

Chapter 14

ABOUT THE DEPARTMENT OF PEDIATRIC AND ADOLESCENT MEDICINE, WESTERN MICHIGAN UNIVERSITY HOMER STRYKER MD SCHOOL OF MEDICINE (WMED), KALAMAZOO, MICHIGAN USA

Mission and service

The Western Michigan University Homer Stryker MD School of Medicine was started in 2012 and its first class of medical students began in 2014. The Department of Pediatric and Adolescent Medicine has a pediatric residency program which is accredited by the Accreditation Council for Graduate Medical Education (ACGME) in Chicago, Illinois, USA and the current residency program in Pediatrics started in 1990.

The WMED Department of Pediatric and Adolescent Medicine has a commitment to a comprehensive approach to the health and development of the child, adolescent, and the family. The Department has a blend of academic general pediatricians and pediatric specialists. Our Pediatric Clinic team provides a broad spectrum of general well and sick child care (birth through 18 years) including immunizations, monitoring general physical and emotional growth, motor skill development, sports medicine (including participation evaluations and evaluation of common sports injuries), child abuse evaluations, and psychosocial or behavioral assessment. WMED Pediatrics believes in immunizations as a protection against preventative disease processes. Our Pediatrics Clinic is undergoing a transformation to a patient-centered medical home (PCMH). A patient-centered medical home is a way to deliver coordinated and comprehensive primary care to our infants, children, adolescents and young adults. It is a partnership between individuals and families within a health care setting, which allows for a more efficient use of resources and time to improve the quality of outcomes for all involved through care provided by a continuity care team.

Research activities

The Department has a variety of research projects in adolescent medicine, neurobehavioral pediatrics, adolescent gynecology, pediatric diabetes mellitus, asthma, and cystic fibrosis. The

WMED Department of Pediatric and Adolescent Medicine has published a number of medical textbooks: Essential adolescent medicine (McGraw-Hill Medical Publishers), The pediatric diagnostic examination (McGraw-Hill), Pediatric and adolescent psychopharmacology (Cambridge University Press), Behavioral pediatrics, 2nd edition (iUniverse Publishers in New York and Lincoln, Nebraska), Behavioral pediatrics 3rd edition (New York: Nova Biomedical Books); 4th Edition: In press. Pediatric practice: Sports medicine (McGraw-Hill), Handbook of clinical pediatrics (Singapore: World Scientific), Neurodevelopmental disabilities: Clinical care for children and young adults (Dordrecht: Springer), Adolescent medicine: Pharmacotherapeutics in medical disorders (Berlin/Boston: De Gruyter), Adolescent medicine: Pharmacotherapeutics in general, mental, and sexual health (Berlin/Boston: De Gruyter), Pediatric psychodermatology (Berlin/Boston: De Gruyter), Substance abuse in adolescents and young adults: A manual for pediatric and primary care clinicians (Berlin/Boston: De Gruyter), and tropical pediatrics (New York: Nova); Second edition in press.

The Department has edited a number of journal issues published by Elsevier Publishers covering pulmonology (State of the Art Reviews: Adolescent Medicine—AM:STARS), genetic disorders in adolescents (AM:STARS), neurologic/neurodevelopmental disorders (AM:STARS), behavioral pediatrics (Pediatric Clinics of North America), pediatric psychopharmacology in the 21st century (Pediatric Clinic of North America), nephrologic disorders in adolescents (AM:STARS), college health (Pediatric Clinics of North America), adolescent medicine (Primary Care: Clinics in Office Practice), behavioral pediatrics in children and adolescents (Primary Care: Clinics in Office Practice), adolescents and sports (Pediatric Clinics of North America), and developmental disabilities (Pediatric Clinics of North America). The Department has also edited a journal issue on musculoskeletal disorders in children and adolescents for the American Academy of Pediatrics' AM:STARs; in April of 2013 a Subspecialty Update issue was published in AM:STARs.

The department has developed academic ties with a variety of international medical centers and organizations, including the Queen Elizabeth Hospital in Hong Kong, Indian Academy of Pediatrics (New Delhi, India), the University of Athens Children's Hospital (First and Second Departments of Paediatrics) in Athens, Greece and the National Institute of Child Health and Human Development in Jerusalem, Israel.

Contact

Professor Donald E Greydanus, MD and Professor Dilip R. Patel, MD
Department of Pediatric and Adolescent Medicine
Western Michigan University Homer Stryker MD School of Medicine
1000 Oakland Drive, D48G, Kalamazoo, MI 49008-1284, United States
E-mail: Donald.greydanus@med.wmich.edu and dilip.Patel@med.wmich.edu
Website: http://www.med.wmich.edu

In: Mental and Holistic Health: Some International Perspectives   ISBN: 978-1-63483-589-3
Editors: J. Calles Jr., D. Greydanus and J. Merrick   © 2015 Nova Science Publishers, Inc.

Chapter 15

ABOUT THE NATIONAL INSTITUTE OF CHILD HEALTH AND HUMAN DEVELOPMENT IN ISRAEL

The National Institute of Child Health and Human Development (NICHD) in Israel was established in 1998 as a virtual institute under the auspicies of the Medical Director, Ministry of Social Affairs and Social Services in order to function as the research arm for the Office of the Medical Director. In 1998 the National Council for Child Health and Pediatrics, Ministry of Health and in 1999 the Director General and Deputy Director General of the Ministry of Health endorsed the establishment of the NICHD.

Mission

The mission of a National Institute for Child Health and Human Development in Israel is to provide an academic focal point for the scholarly interdisciplinary study of child life, health, public health, welfare, disability, rehabilitation, intellectual disability and related aspects of human development. This mission includes research, teaching, clinical work, information and public service activities in the field of child health and human development.

Service and academic activities

Over the years many activities became focused in the south of Israel due to collaboration with various professionals at the Faculty of Health Sciences (FOHS) at the Ben Gurion University of the Negev (BGU). Since 2000 an affiliation with the Zusman Child Development Center at the Pediatric Division of Soroka University Medical Center has resulted in collaboration around the establishment of the Down Syndrome Clinic at that center. In 2002 a full course on "Disability" was established at the Recanati School for Allied Professions in the Community, FOHS, and BGU and in 2005 collaboration was started with the Primary Care Unit of the faculty and disability became part of the master of public health course on "Children and society." In the academic year 2005-2006 a one semester course on "Aging with disability" was started as part of the master of science program in gerontology in our collaboration with the Center for Multidisciplinary Research in Aging. In 2010 collaborations with the Division of Pediatrics, Hadassah Hebrew University Medical Center, Jerusalem, Israel around the National Down Syndrome Center and teaching students and residents about intellectual and developmental disabilities as part of their training at this campus.

Research activities

The affiliated staff has over the years published work from projects and research activities in this national and international collaboration. In the year 2000 the International Journal of Adolescent Medicine and Health and in 2005 the International Journal on Disability and Human Development of De Gruyter Publishing House (Berlin and New York) were affiliated with the National Institute of Child Health and Human Development. From 2008 also the International Journal of Child Health and Human Development (Nova Science, New York), the International Journal of Child and Adolescent Health (Nova Science) and the Journal of Pain Management (Nova Science) affiliated and from 2009 the International Public Health Journal (Nova Science) and Journal of Alternative Medicine Research (Nova Science). All peer-reviewed international journals.

National collaborations

Nationally the NICHD works in collaboration with the Faculty of Health Sciences, Ben Gurion University of the Negev; Department of Physical Therapy, Sackler School of Medicine, Tel Aviv University; Autism Center, Assaf HaRofeh Medical Center; National Rett and PKU Centers at Chaim Sheba Medical Center, Tel HaShomer; Department of Physiotherapy, Haifa University; Department of Education, Bar Ilan University, Ramat Gan, Faculty of Social Sciences and Health Sciences; College of Judea and Samaria in Ariel and in 2011 affiliation with Center for Pediatric Chronic Diseases and National Center for Down Syndrome, Department of Pediatrics, Hadassah Hebrew University Medical Center, Mount Scopus Campus, Jerusalem.

International collaborations

Internationally with the Department of Disability and Human Development, College of Applied Health Sciences, University of Illinois at Chicago; Strong Center for Developmental Disabilities, Golisano Children's Hospital at Strong, University of Rochester School of Medicine and Dentistry, New York; Centre on Intellectual Disabilities, University of Albany, New York; Centre for Chronic Disease Prevention and Control, Health Canada, Ottawa; Chandler Medical Center and Children's Hospital, Kentucky Children's Hospital, Section of Adolescent Medicine, University of Kentucky, Lexington; Chronic Disease Prevention and Control Research Center, Baylor College of Medicine, Houston, Texas; Division of Neuroscience, Department of Psychiatry, Columbia University, New York; Institute for the Study of Disadvantage and Disability, Atlanta; Center for Autism and Related Disorders, Department Psychiatry, Children's Hospital Boston, Boston; Department of Pediatric and Adolescent Medicine, Western Michigan University Homer Stryker MD School of Medicine,

Kalamazoo, Michigan, United States; Department of Paediatrics, Child Health and Adolescent Medicine, Children's Hospital at Westmead, Westmead, Australia; International Centre for the Study of Occupational and Mental Health, Düsseldorf, Germany; Centre for Advanced Studies in Nursing, Department of General Practice and Primary Care, University of Aberdeen, Aberdeen, United Kingdom; Quality of Life Research Center, Copenhagen, Denmark; Nordic School of Public Health, Gottenburg, Sweden, Scandinavian Institute of Quality of Working Life, Oslo, Norway; The Department of Applied Social Sciences (APSS) of The Hong Kong Polytechnic University Hong Kong.

Targets

Our focus is on research, international collaborations, clinical work, teaching and policy in health, disability and human development and to establish the NICHD as a permanent institute at one of the residential care centers for persons with intellectual disability in Israel in order to conduct model research and together with the four university schools of public health/medicine in Israel establish a national master and doctoral program in disability and human development at the institute to secure the next generation of professionals working in this often non-prestigious/low-status field of work.

Contact

Joav Merrick, MD, MMedSci, DMSc
Professor of Pediatrics
Medical Director, Health Services, Division for Intellectual and Developmental Disabilities, Ministry of Social Affairs and Social Services, POB 1260, IL-91012 Jerusalem, Israel.
E-mail: jmerrick@zahav.net.il

In: Mental and Holistic Health: Some International Perspectives   ISBN: 978-1-63483-589-3
Editors: J. Calles Jr., D. Greydanus and J. Merrick   © 2015 Nova Science Publishers, Inc.

Chapter 16

ABOUT THE BOOK SERIES "HEALTH AND HUMAN DEVELOPMENT"

Health and human development is a book series with publications from a multidisciplinary group of researchers, practitioners and clinicians for an international professional forum interested in the broad spectrum of health and human development. Books already published:

- Merrick J, Omar HA, eds. Adolescent behavior research. International perspectives. New York: Nova Science, 2007.
- Kratky KW. Complementary medicine systems: Comparison and integration. New York: Nova Science, 2008.
- Schofield P, Merrick J, eds. Pain in children and youth. New York: Nova Science, 2009.
- Greydanus DE, Patel DR, Pratt HD, Calles Jr JL, eds. Behavioral pediatrics, 3 ed. New York: Nova Science, 2009.
- Ventegodt S, Merrick J, eds. Meaningful work: Research in quality of working life. New York: Nova Science, 2009.
- Omar HA, Greydanus DE, Patel DR, Merrick J, eds. Obesity and adolescence. A public health concern. New York: Nova Science, 2009.
- Lieberman A, Merrick J, eds. Poverty and children. A public health concern. New York: Nova Science, 2009.
- Goodbread J. Living on the edge. The mythical, spiritual and philosophical roots of social marginality. New York: Nova Science, 2009.
- Bennett DL, Towns S, Elliot E, Merrick J, eds. Challenges in adolescent health: An Australian perspective. New York: Nova Science, 2009.
- Schofield P, Merrick J, eds. Children and pain. New York: Nova Science, 2009.
- Sher L, Kandel I, Merrick J, eds. Alcohol-related cognitive disorders: Research and clinical perspectives. New York: Nova Science, 2009.
- Anyanwu EC. Advances in environmental health effects of toxigenic mold and mycotoxins. New York: Nova Science, 2009.
- Bell E, Merrick J, eds. Rural child health. International aspects. New York: Nova Science, 2009.
- Dubowitz H, Merrick J, eds. International aspects of child abuse and neglect. New York: Nova Science, 2010.

- Shahtahmasebi S, Berridge D. Conceptualizing behavior: A practical guide to data analysis. New York: Nova Science, 2010.
- Wernik U. Chance action and therapy. The playful way of changing. New York: Nova Science, 2010.
- Omar HA, Greydanus DE, Patel DR, Merrick J, eds. Adolescence and chronic illness. A public health concern. New York: Nova Science, 2010.
- Patel DR, Greydanus DE, Omar HA, Merrick J, eds. Adolescence and sports. New York: Nova Science, 2010.
- Shek DTL, Ma HK, Merrick J, eds. Positive youth development: Evaluation and future directions in a Chinese context. New York: Nova Science, 2010.
- Shek DTL, Ma HK, Merrick J, eds. Positive youth development: Implementation of a youth program in a Chinese context. New York: Nova Science, 2010.
- Omar HA, Greydanus DE, Tsitsika AK, Patel DR, Merrick J, eds. Pediatric and adolescent sexuality and gynecology: Principles for the primary care clinician. New York: Nova Science, 2010.
- Chow E, Merrick J, eds. Advanced cancer. Pain and quality of life. New York: Nova Science, 2010.
- Latzer Y, Merrick, J, Stein D, eds. Understanding eating disorders. Integrating culture, psychology and biology. New York: Nova Science, 2010.
- Sahgal A, Chow E, Merrick J, eds. Bone and brain metastases: Advances in research and treatment. New York: Nova Science, 2010.
- Postolache TT, Merrick J, eds. Environment, mood disorders and suicide. New York: Nova Science, 2010.
- Maharajh HD, Merrick J, eds. Social and cultural psychiatry experience from the Caribbean Region. New York: Nova Science, 2010.
- Mirsky J. Narratives and meanings of migration. New York: Nova Science, 2010.
- Harvey PW. Self-management and the health care consumer. New York: Nova Science, 2011.
- Ventegodt S, Merrick J. Sexology from a holistic point of view. New York: Nova Science, 2011.
- Ventegodt S, Merrick J. Principles of holistic psychiatry: A textbook on holistic medicine for mental disorders. New York: Nova Science, 2011.
- Greydanus DE, Calles Jr JL, Patel DR, Nazeer A, Merrick J, eds. Clinical aspects of psychopharmacology in childhood and adolescence. New York: Nova Science, 2011.
- Bell E, Seidel BM, Merrick J, eds. Climate change and rural child health. New York: Nova Science, 2011.
- Bell E, Zimitat C, Merrick J, eds. Rural medical education: Practical strategies. New York: Nova Science, 2011.
- Latzer Y, Tzischinsky. The dance of sleeping and eating among adolescents: Normal and pathological perspectives. New York: Nova Science, 2011.
- Deshmukh VD. The astonishing brain and holistic consciousness: Neuroscience and Vedanta perspectives. New York: Nova Science, 2011.
- Bell E, Westert GP, Merrick J, eds. Translational research for primary healthcare. New York: Nova Science, 2011.
- Shek DTL, Sun RCF, Merrick J, eds. Drug abuse in Hong Kong: Development and evaluation of a prevention program. New York: Nova Science, 2011.
- Ventegodt S, Hermansen TD, Merrick J. Human Development: Biology from a holistic point of view. New York: Nova Science, 2011.

- Ventegodt S, Merrick J. Our search for meaning in life. New York: Nova Science, 2011.
- Caron RM, Merrick J, eds. Building community capacity: Minority and immigrant populations. New York: Nova Science, 2012.
- Klein H, Merrick J, eds. Human immunodeficiency virus (HIV) research: Social science aspects. New York: Nova Science, 2012.
- Lutzker JR, Merrick J, eds. Applied public health: Examining multifaceted Social or ecological problems and child maltreatment. New York: Nova Science, 2012.
- Chemtob D, Merrick J, eds. AIDS and tuberculosis: Public health aspects. New York: Nova Science, 2012.
- Ventegodt S, Merrick J. Textbook on evidence-based holistic mind-body medicine: Basic principles of healing in traditional Hippocratic medicine. New York: Nova Science, 2012.
- Ventegodt S, Merrick J. Textbook on evidence-based holistic mind-body medicine: Holistic practice of traditional Hippocratic medicine. New York: Nova Science, 2012.
- Ventegodt S, Merrick J. Textbook on evidence-based holistic mind-body medicine: Healing the mind in traditional Hippocratic medicine. New York: Nova Science, 2012.
- Ventegodt S, Merrick J. Textbook on evidence-based holistic mind-body medicine: Sexology and traditional Hippocratic medicine. New York: Nova Science, 2012.
- Ventegodt S, Merrick J. Textbook on evidence-based holistic mind-body medicine: Research, philosophy, economy and politics of traditional Hippocratic medicine. New York: Nova Science, 2012.
- Caron RM, Merrick J, eds. Building community capacity: Skills and principles. New York: Nova Science, 2012.
- Lemal M, Merrick J, eds. Health risk communication. New York: Nova Science, 2012.
- Ventegodt S, Merrick J. Textbook on evidence-based holistic mind-body medicine: Basic philosophy and ethics of traditional Hippocratic medicine. New York: Nova Science, 2013.
- Caron RM, Merrick J, eds. Building community capacity: Case examples from around the world. New York: Nova Science, 2013.
- Steele RE. Managed care in a public setting. New York: Nova Science, 2013.
- Srabstein JC, Merrick J, eds. Bullying: A public health concern. New York: Nova Science, 2013.
- Pulenzas N, Lechner B, Thavarajah N, Chow E, Merrick J, eds. Advanced cancer: Managing symptoms and quality of life. New York: Nova Science, 2013.
- Stein D, Latzer Y, eds. Treatment and recovery of eating disorders. New York: Nova Science, 2013.
- Sun J, Buys N, Merrick J. Health promotion: Community singing as a vehicle to promote health. New York: Nova Science, 2013.
- Pulenzas N, Lechner B, Thavarajah N, Chow E, Merrick J, eds. Advanced cancer: Managing symptoms and quality of life. New York: Nova Science, 2013.
- Sun J, Buys N, Merrick J. Health promotion: Strengthening positive health and preventing disease. New York: Nova Science, 2013.
- Merrick J, Israeli S, eds. Food, nutrition and eating behavior. New York: Nova Science, 2013.
- Shahtahmasebi S, Merrick J. Suicide from a public health perspective.
  New York: Nova Science, 2014.
- Merrick J, Tenenbaum A, eds. Public health concern: Smoking, alcohol and substance use. New York: Nova Science, 2014.

- Merrick J, Aspler S, Morad M, eds. Mental health from an international perspective. New York: Nova Science, 2014.
- Merrick J, ed. India: Health and human development aspects. New York: Nova Science, 2014.
- Caron R, Merrick J, eds. Public health: Improving health via inter-professional collaborations. New York: Nova Science, 2014.
- Merrick J, ed. Pain Mangement Yearbook 2014. New York: Nova Science, 2015.
- Merrick J, ed. Public Health Yearbook 2014. New York: Nova Science, 2015.
- Sher L, Merrick J, eds. Forensic psychiatry: A public health perspective. New York: Nova Science, 2015.
- Shek DTL, Wu FKY, Merrick J, eds. Leadership and service learning education: Holistic development for Chinese university students. New York: Nova Science, 2015.

Contact

Professor Joav Merrick, MD, MMedSci, DMSc
Medical Director, Health Services
Division for Intellectual and Developmental Disabailities
Ministry of Social Affairs and Social Services
POBox 1260, IL-91012 Jerusalem, Israel
E-mail: jmerrick@zahav.net.il

Section Four: Index

INDEX

#

504, 100

A

abuse, 16, 32, 46, 53, 66, 78, 83, 91, 99, 166, 172, 174, 180
academic difficulties, 91
academic learning, 15
academic performance, 63
academic problems, 94
adolescents, xi, 5, 6, 12, 13, 15, 16, 20, 26, 27, 29, 30, 31, 32, 34, 35, 39, 41, 49, 52, 56, 57, 59, 60, 61, 63, 65, 66, 67, 68, 70, 71, 72, 73, 75, 76, 77, 84, 86, 87, 88, 89, 90, 91, 92, 93, 94, 96, 97, 99, 100, 102, 103, 114, 115, 158, 173, 174, 180
adulthood, 5, 11, 34, 44, 56, 63, 77, 97, 107
adults, 5, 13, 32, 54, 60, 62, 68, 73, 81, 86, 87, 88, 89, 94, 100, 106, 107, 113, 130, 174
Africa, 163, 164, 165, 166, 167
aggressive behavior, 35, 37, 41, 42, 44, 45, 46, 47, 48, 49, 50, 51, 52, 53, 54, 77, 82
agoraphobia, 34, 95, 97
AIDS, 5, 164, 165, 181
alcohol abuse, 65, 97
alcohol dependence, 34, 38, 48
alcohol problems, 48, 53
alcohol use, 16, 38
alkaloids, 158, 159, 160
alternative medicine, 135, 137, 139, 140
American Psychiatric Association, 25, 30, 38, 50, 57, 72, 88, 89, 103, 114
amphetamines, 16, 21, 65
anger, 14, 24, 29, 30, 42, 43, 44, 45, 47, 48, 49, 50, 53, 151, 154
antidepressant, 24, 51, 52, 55, 59, 67, 68, 70, 72, 83, 90, 102, 115

antidepressant medication, 59, 67, 68, 70, 72
antidepressants, 24, 51, 54, 68, 73, 99, 101, 102, 120, 130
antipsychotic, 6, 52, 54, 55, 71, 89, 120, 125, 128
antipsychotic drugs, 120, 125
antisocial behavior, 44
antisocial personality disorder, 16, 46, 50
anxiety, xi, 12, 18, 19, 24, 34, 46, 47, 50, 51, 52, 54, 55, 57, 63, 65, 73, 76, 79, 80, 84, 90, 91, 93, 94, 95, 96, 97, 98, 99, 100, 101, 102, 103, 106, 108, 109, 110, 111, 112, 159
anxiety disorder, xi, 18, 19, 34, 46, 50, 65, 73, 76, 79, 84, 91, 93, 94, 95, 96, 97, 98, 99, 100, 102, 103, 106, 108, 112, 159
anxiety disorder due to another medical condition, 96
aripiprazole, 37, 53, 55, 89
Aristotle, 4, 6
assessment, 11, 20, 26, 35, 39, 41, 47, 49, 56, 61, 78, 88, 97, 98, 103, 105, 106, 107, 110, 114
asthma, 99, 173
attention deficit hyperactivity disorder, (ADHD), 6, 11, 12, 13, 14, 15, 16, 17, 18, 19, 20, 21, 22, 23, 24, 25, 26, 27, 34, 35, 36, 38, 47, 48, 49, 50, 52, 53, 54, 55, 57, 62, 66, 68, 76, 79, 80, 81, 83, 85, 90, 97, 108, 109
avoidance, 62, 94, 95, 96, 97, 110
avoidance behavior, 110

B

basal ganglia, 107
behavior therapy, 92, 93, 99, 115
behavioral assessment, 51, 173
behaviors, xi, 12, 13, 14, 15, 16, 19, 30, 31, 32, 33, 35, 36, 41, 42, 43, 45, 47, 48, 49, 56, 57, 63, 66, 91, 94, 97, 99, 102, 106, 107, 109, 110, 111, 112
benzodiazepines, 83, 84, 99, 101

bipolar disorder, xi, 18, 34, 50, 51, 71, 75, 76, 77, 78, 79, 81, 82, 84, 86, 87, 88, 89, 90, 91, 92, 112, 120
black box warning, 83, 102, 112
borderline personality disorder, 50
Botswana, xii, 163, 165
bowel, 64
brain, 17, 46, 47, 51, 64, 77, 79, 143, 180
Brazil, 159, 160
bullying, 63, 98
Buspirone, 55, 84, 101

C

Canabis sativa, 6
cancer, 125, 129, 130, 137, 138, 149, 180, 181
cannabis, 48, 50, 65
Caribbean, 2, 180
CDC, 43, 48
central nervous system (CNS), 16, 48, 65, 73, 99, 159
chemotherapy, 17, 120, 121, 128
Chicago, 75, 172, 173, 176
child abuse, 173, 179
Child Behavior Checklist, 115
child maltreatment, 181
childhood, 5, 14, 26, 30, 38, 47, 56, 57, 73, 78, 84, 87, 88, 89, 90, 91, 93, 96, 97, 99, 102, 103, 105, 106, 114, 115, 151, 180
childhood aggression, 57
chromosome(s), 10, 114
citalopram, 68, 70, 101, 112, 113
clinical holistic medicine, 139, 140
clinical presentation, 60, 75, 79, 87, 108
clinical syndrome, 114
clinical trials, 67, 100, 130, 156
Clonazepam, 91, 101
cognitive impairment(s), 79
cognitive-behavioral therapy (CBT), 59, 67, 68, 72, 84, 86, 91, 92, 93, 99, 100, 102, 110, 111, 112, 113, 115
collaboration, 106, 120, 122, 125, 137, 175, 176
comorbid diagnoses, 83
comorbidity, 11, 20, 25, 35, 38, 47, 50, 63, 66, 72, 73, 88, 90, 98, 106, 107, 110, 111, 115
compulsive behavior, 106, 109, 110, 111
compulsive personality disorder, 109
conduct disorder, xi, 16, 18, 29, 30, 37, 38, 39, 47, 49, 56, 66
consciousness, 139, 144, 145, 146, 150, 151, 152, 155, 160, 180
Controlled Substances Act, 158
controlled trials, 27, 39, 68, 84, 86, 99, 113, 130, 139
controversial, 71, 107

coronary heart disease, 125, 131, 138, 140
Council of Europe, 129, 131

D

Department of Education, 176
Department of Health and Human Services, 43
depression, 18, 19, 24, 47, 49, 50, 51, 54, 57, 59, 60, 61, 62, 63, 64, 65, 66, 67, 68, 71, 72, 73, 75, 76, 77, 79, 81, 82, 86, 87, 89, 90, 97, 98, 100, 102, 112, 130, 145, 149, 151, 157
depressive symptoms, 61, 62, 65, 80
developmental disorder, 34, 55, 171
diabetes, 5, 17, 64, 65, 73, 82, 173
Diagnostic and statistical manual, 5th edition (DSM-5), 12, 15, 25, 30, 34, 50, 60, 62, 76, 94, 95, 96, 106, 108, 109
diagnostic criteria, 11, 30, 60, 61, 78, 109
Digitalis purpurea, 6
disorder, xi, 6, 11, 12, 15, 17, 18, 19, 24, 25, 26, 27, 29, 30, 31, 32, 33, 34, 35, 36, 38, 39, 46, 47, 49, 50, 51, 52, 53, 54, 55, 57, 60, 63, 64, 65, 66, 72, 75, 76, 78, 79, 83, 84, 86, 87, 88, 89, 90, 91, 94, 95, 96, 97, 99, 100, 105, 106, 107, 108, 109, 110, 113, 114, 115, 116
disposition, 146, 159
distress, 24, 59, 62, 63, 64, 79, 94, 95, 97, 99, 106, 107, 110
dizygotic twins, 107
dizziness, 113
doctors, 119, 120, 123, 125, 137, 142, 157, 166
dosage, 21, 68, 70, 71
dosing, 51, 68, 70, 71, 85, 113, 158
Down syndrome, 66
drug interaction, 81
drug treatment, 124, 125
drugs, 3, 5, 6, 16, 17, 48, 51, 89, 99, 113, 119, 120, 121, 122, 123, 125, 126, 128, 129, 131, 132, 135, 136, 137, 139, 140, 141, 143, 145, 147
duloxetine, 68, 70, 101, 103
dysphoria, 59, 72
dysthymia, 73
dysthymic disorder, xi, 59, 60

E

eating disorders, 180, 181
ECG, 113
ecstasy, 153
education, 7, 14, 86, 87, 135, 138, 171, 180, 182
EEG, 51, 98
Egypt, 4

EKG, 98
emotional disorder, 98, 103
emotional distress, 62
emotional problems, 103
emotional responses, 93
emotional state, 48, 49
empathy, 30, 32
encephalitis, 47, 51, 56
endocrine disorders, 99
energy, 29, 60, 63, 65, 98, 99, 124, 137, 148, 149, 150, 151, 152, 153, 155, 156
England, 5, 6, 7
enuresis, 18, 108
environment, 4, 44, 45, 63, 79, 87
environmental factors, 97
environmental issues, 67
environmental stress, 49
Ephedra, 3
epidemic, 61, 72, 167
epidemiologic, 88
epidemiologic studies, 88
epidemiology, 25, 30, 38, 41, 88, 89, 105, 106
epilepsy, 4, 47, 52, 56, 57, 64, 65, 73
Epstein-Barr virus, 17, 64
Erythroxylon coca, 6
escitalopram, 54, 55, 68, 70, 84, 101, 112, 113
ethics, 130, 140, 160, 163, 164, 166, 167, 181
etiology, 5, 50, 87, 96, 105, 107
Europe, 4, 5
European Commission, 128
evolution, 16, 145, 150
examinations, 122, 126
executive function, 27, 79, 83, 158
external locus of control, 86
externalizing behavior, 39, 54, 98
externalizing disorders, 47, 99

F

family functioning, 76, 86
family history, 25, 78, 79, 107, 110
family members, 13, 19, 31, 41, 44, 51, 63, 110
family system, 86
family therapy, 87, 100
family violence, 57
FDA approval, 24, 100, 112, 113
fear(s), 30, 44, 93, 94, 95, 97, 99, 100, 108, 109, 110, 115, 132, 146, 151, 154, 155, 164
fear hierarchy, 100
feelings, 29, 42, 43, 52, 63, 65, 98, 135, 137, 138, 151, 152, 154, 155
fetal alcohol syndrome (FAS), 52, 55
fibrosis, 64, 174

fluoxetine, 54, 55, 67, 68, 70, 91, 100, 101, 112, 113
fluvoxamine, 91, 100, 101, 112, 113
food, 13, 14, 20, 21, 22, 23, 84, 85, 94, 144, 147
Food and Drug Administration (FDA), 6, 22, 24, 67, 68, 71, 80, 81, 100, 101, 112, 113
fractures, 14, 70, 124
fragments, 153

G

generalized anxiety disorder, 19, 84, 95, 96, 103, 108
genetic disorders, 174
genetic factors, 44, 107
Georgia, 172
Germany, 5, 6, 140, 177
gerontology, 175
God, 144
Greece, 4, 171, 174
guidance, 44, 49, 131, 155
guidelines, 51, 68, 85, 91, 112
guilt, 30, 108, 109

H

hallucinations, 50, 78, 128, 146
happiness, 136, 154, 166
healing, xii, 130, 136, 140, 141, 142, 143, 144, 145, 147, 148, 149, 150, 152, 153, 154, 155, 156, 157, 158, 159, 160, 161, 163, 164, 165, 181
health problems, 120, 128
health services, 97
health status, 90
heart attack, 95
heart disease, 17
heart failure, 5
heart rate, 23
heavy drinking, 48
helplessness, 63
herbal medicine, 135, 137
heterogeneity, 76, 79
high blood pressure, 82
high school, 16, 48
HIV, 5, 17, 64, 164, 165, 181
holistic medicine, 129, 139, 142, 156, 157, 180
Hong Kong, 4, 174, 177, 180
hopelessness, 60, 63, 86, 159
human development, xii, 172, 175, 177, 179, 182
hyperactivity, xi, 6, 11, 12, 13, 14, 15, 16, 18, 24, 25, 26, 27, 33, 34, 38, 39, 46, 47, 55, 57, 66, 76, 79, 89, 90, 91, 108
hyperactivity-impulsivity, 12
hyperarousal, 84, 85

I

hyperparathyroidism, 99
hypersensitivity, 20
hypersomnia, 60
hypertension, 23
hyperthyroidism, 85, 99
hypnosis, 25
hypomania, 76, 78
hypotension, 23, 24

I

idiopathic, 85, 90
impairments, 35, 46, 47, 52, 53, 63, 76, 79, 89, 105
imprisonment, 165
improvements, 86
impulsive, 15, 16, 34, 45, 49, 57, 78
impulsivity, 13, 14, 15, 16, 18, 19, 34, 38, 45, 49, 75
in utero, 107
inattention, 12, 14, 16, 18, 79, 83
incidence, 52, 61, 106, 107
income, 164
India, 7, 171, 174, 182
Individualized Education Program (IEP), 100
individuals, 30, 45, 49, 52, 60, 98, 108, 109, 173
infants, 62, 93, 94, 173
infection, 17, 107, 108, 110, 113, 164
influenza, 120, 121, 128, 130, 131, 132, 133
influenza vaccine, 120, 128
inhibition, 97, 159
inhibitor, 21, 22, 24, 68, 83, 100, 116, 142
insomnia, 24, 60, 65, 85, 90
integration, 156, 179
intelligence, 7, 49
intelligence scores, 7
internalizing, 39, 98
interpersonal conflict, 44, 87
interpersonal relations, 11
interpersonal relationships, 11
intervention, 36, 43, 51, 53, 73, 75, 83, 84, 86, 87, 111, 114
intoxication, 46, 48, 66
irradiation, 17
irritability, 14, 24, 26, 47, 48, 49, 52, 53, 54, 62, 65, 66, 70, 73, 75, 76, 78, 80, 96, 101, 110
isolation, 33, 62, 63, 77, 100

J

juvenile delinquents, 6, 31
juveniles, 73

K

kill, 128, 149, 166
kindergarten, 94

L

language skills, 44
learning, 18, 79, 89, 99, 101, 111, 142, 145, 152, 156, 182
lifestyle changes, 131, 140
Limpopo, 164, 165
lithium, 52, 53, 54, 55, 57, 71, 72, 80, 81, 82, 84, 85, 89
longitudinal study, 38
Lorazepam, 101
loss of consciousness, 156
love, 138, 153, 154, 155, 166, 167
LSD, 141, 142, 148, 153, 154, 156, 157
lupus erythematosus, 64

M

major depression, 76
major depressive disorder, 34, 60, 73, 89, 95
management, 5, 6, 25, 35, 41, 44, 56, 73, 75, 83, 84, 85, 86, 87, 89, 100, 101, 102, 180
mania, 24, 50, 51, 54, 76, 78, 80, 81, 83, 84, 86, 88, 89, 90
manic, 50, 80, 84, 89, 90, 101, 112, 115
manic episode, 80, 112
manipulation, 25, 124
marijuana, 6, 48, 65, 99
MAS, 21, 23, 53, 55
masturbation, 4
matter, x, 70, 71, 122, 123, 146, 155
Mauritius, 37
medical, 4, 5, 6, 7, 18, 19, 20, 25, 27, 29, 37, 41, 43, 46, 47, 50, 51, 52, 53, 56, 63, 65, 73, 96, 98, 99, 110, 122, 125, 126, 143, 144, 145, 149, 157, 160, 165, 171, 172, 173, 174, 180
medicinal herbs, 3
medicine, xi, 4, 5, 7, 119, 120, 121, 122, 124, 125, 126, 128, 129, 130, 131, 135, 136, 137, 138, 139, 140, 141, 142, 144, 145, 146, 148, 149, 156, 157, 160, 165, 166, 172, 173, 174, 177, 179, 181
melatonin, 55, 83, 85
mellitus, 5, 17, 64, 65, 82, 173
memory, 65, 79, 101, 143, 150
mental disorder, 12, 25, 30, 38, 60, 72, 88, 95, 103, 114, 124, 156, 157, 180
mental health, 4, 6, 27, 78, 96, 98, 99, 102, 122, 128

mental retardation, 49
meta-analysis, 26, 114, 122, 130, 140
metabolic disorder(s), 107
metabolic syndrome, 82
metabolism, 68
methamphetamine, 21, 48, 65, 99
methodology, 122
methylphenidate, 6, 21, 23, 53, 54, 55, 57, 83
mind-body, 25, 130, 131, 139, 140, 156, 160, 181
Mirtazapine, 70, 101
mnemonic processes, 88
modifications, 62, 143
mold, 5, 179
molecules, 155
monoamine oxidase inhibitors, 71
mood disorder, 34, 49, 54, 57, 78, 92, 171, 180
mood stabilization, 80
mood states, 76, 79
mood swings, 77
morbidity, 47, 88, 114
mortality, 47, 128
mortality rate, 128
musculoskeletal, 174
mushrooms, 4, 148
mystical experiences, 145

N

narcolepsy, 24, 132
narratives, 19, 56
National Health and Nutrition Examination Survey (NHANES), 61
National Institute of Mental Health, 109
nausea, 82, 101, 149
NCS, 96, 103
negative consequences, 32, 33, 45
negative effects, 62, 122, 123, 125, 126
neurodegenerative disorders, 160
neurodevelopmental disorders, 174
Nobel Prize, 172
norepinephrine, 22, 68, 83, 100
normal development, 31, 33
North America, 159, 174
Norway, 141, 163, 177
nutrition, 39, 181

O

observable behavior, 33
observed behavior, 35
obsessive-compulsive disorder, 50, 114, 115

OCD, 96, 100, 102, 105, 106, 107, 108, 109, 110, 111, 112, 113, 114, 115
ODD, 18, 29, 30, 31, 32, 33, 34, 35, 36, 37, 38, 49, 50, 53, 66, 76, 79, 97
olanzapine, 37, 80
opiates, 17
organ(s), 150, 163, 164, 165, 166
organised crime, 130, 139
other specified anxiety disorder, 96

P

panic attack(s), 95, 96
panic disorder, 65, 95, 97
panic symptoms, 98
parents, 12, 13, 14, 15, 18, 25, 29, 31, 32, 33, 36, 61, 62, 63, 67, 68, 77, 78, 79, 80, 84, 86, 99, 100, 106, 107, 108, 110, 112, 151
paroxetine, 68, 70, 100, 101, 112, 113
participants, 144, 145, 157, 160
pathogenesis, 67, 79, 107
pathologist, 5, 53
pathology, 19
PCP, 66
pediatrician, 29, 35, 38, 41, 47
peer rejection, 45, 49, 57
peer relationship, 67, 86
pelvic floor, 130
pelvis, 147, 148
personal development, 142, 145, 146
personality, 12, 46, 50, 54, 87, 109, 145, 146, 160
personality disorder(s), 12, 46, 50, 54
personality traits, 87, 160
Peru, xii, 141, 142, 143, 146, 157, 158
pharmaceutical, 6, 7, 119, 120, 121, 122, 123, 124, 125, 126, 128, 129, 131, 136, 139, 140
pharmacogenetics, 57
pharmacokinetics, 159
pharmacologic agents, 4, 53
pharmacological treatment, 80, 85
pharmacology, 4, 5, 6, 7, 143, 159
pharmacopoeia, 4
pharmacotherapy, 21, 27, 35, 39, 52, 54, 59, 72, 73, 75, 80, 86, 87, 90, 91, 100, 103, 111
phenomenology, 57, 88
phenotype(s), 88, 91
phenytoin, 54, 55
Philadelphia, 90, 114
phobia, 94, 96
PKU, 176
placebo, 6, 27, 37, 54, 57, 67, 68, 89, 90, 91, 100, 101, 102, 103, 110, 112, 116, 121, 122, 126, 130, 136, 165

post-traumatic stress disorder (PTSD), 50, 95, 96, 97
Prader-Willi syndrome, 46, 48, 52, 55, 110
prednisone, 81
preparation, x, 21, 85, 144, 145, 160
preschool, 13, 14, 19, 26, 31, 32, 38, 56, 72, 90, 94
preschool children, 26, 32, 38, 56, 72
principles, 4, 7, 35, 80, 84, 111, 125, 130, 140, 160, 181
problem solving, 75, 79, 80, 86, 87
prodrome, 65
professionals, 26, 175, 177
prognosis, 18, 51, 65, 108, 109
prolactin, 82
prophylaxis, 90
propranolol, 51, 84, 85
prostate cancer, 131, 140
psychiatric disorder(s), 18, 21, 24, 25, 26, 29, 30, 33, 34, 35, 36, 37, 41, 44, 46, 49, 50, 51, 52, 53, 54, 56, 59, 64, 65, 67, 97, 98, 105, 106, 130, 140
psychiatric illness, 109, 114
psychiatric patients, 137
psychiatrist, 6, 71
psychiatry, 5, 50, 103, 110, 120, 125, 180, 182
psychodynamic psychotherapy, 100, 130, 137, 140
psychoeducational intervention, 86
psychologist, 19, 35
psychology, 86, 136, 140, 180
psychometric properties, 78
psychopathology, 30, 47, 62
psychopharmacology, 7, 57, 143, 159, 171, 174, 180
psychosis, 50, 51, 54, 80, 89, 99, 108, 124
psychosocial functioning, 86
psychosocial impairment, 75, 85, 87
psychosocial interventions, 29, 37, 53, 86
psychosocial therapies, 85
psychosomatic, 125, 156
psychostimulants, 37, 83, 99
psychotherapy, 37, 53, 59, 67, 72, 73, 86, 87, 92, 99, 100, 102, 111, 125, 130, 137, 139, 140
psychotropic drugs, 130, 139
psychotropic medications, 21, 41, 52, 56
public health, 7, 129, 172, 175, 177, 179, 180, 181, 182

Q

QT interval, 82
quality of life, 120, 121, 122, 124, 125, 129, 136, 139, 157, 160, 172, 180, 181
quetiapine, 54, 80, 89

R

rape, 31, 32, 164, 165, 166, 167
rating scale(s), 19, 35, 36, 88, 98, 109
regression analysis, 27
rehabilitation, 172, 175
REM, 83
remorse, 32, 77
renal failure, 17, 64
repetitive behavior, 108, 109
replication, 103
requirement(s), 37, 103, 106
research institutions, 122
researchers, 6, 50, 119, 120, 122, 123, 135, 137, 138, 179
restless legs syndrome, 18
retardation, 60
risk factors, 30, 45, 51
risk-taking, 16, 78
risperidone, 35, 37, 52, 53, 54, 57, 80, 116
robberies, 145
role playing, 87
romantic relationship, 16
routines, 15, 87, 108

S

sadness, 59, 63, 152
salicylates, 5, 6
schizophrenia, 50, 71, 72, 130, 137
school, 12, 13, 14, 15, 19, 29, 30, 32, 33, 35, 39, 41, 43, 44, 49, 62, 63, 66, 77, 79, 83, 86, 90, 91, 92, 94, 96, 99, 100, 106, 108, 109, 110, 177
science, 4, 5, 79, 122, 130, 136, 138, 175, 181
sclerosis, 46, 48, 52, 55
seizure, 44, 47, 51, 52, 53, 55, 57
selective mutism, 94, 96
selective serotonin reuptake inhibitor SSRI(s), 37, 51, 52, 54, 55, 68, 70, 71, 80, 83, 84, 93, 99, 100, 101, 102, 103, 112, 113
self-efficacy, 86
self-esteem, 16, 26, 60, 67, 75, 77, 78, 86
sensitivity, 62, 66, 77, 109, 145
sensory impairments, 47
separation anxiety disorder, 46, 94
serotonin, 52, 67, 71, 73, 100, 112, 113, 116, 143
serotonin syndrome, 71
sertraline, 68, 70, 100, 101, 102, 103, 110, 112, 113, 115
serum, 85, 113
services, x, 123
sex, 6, 33, 78, 147

sexual abuse, 78
sexual problems, 119, 120, 128
sexuality, 4, 135, 137, 138, 180
shamanism, 145, 146
shame, 106, 149, 150, 151, 152
shyness, 95
side effects, 6, 23, 24, 25, 37, 68, 71, 72, 81, 100, 101, 102, 112, 113, 121, 124, 125, 137, 139, 140, 143, 156, 160
sleep disturbance, 80, 90, 98
smallpox, 5
SMS, 52, 55
social anxiety, 50, 94, 95, 99
social anxiety disorder, 19, 46, 95
social context, 44, 48
social impairment, 38, 91, 99
social phobia, 34, 95, 97, 102
social situations, 50, 95
social skills, 26, 86
socialization, 16, 49
society, 132, 165, 175
sodium, 81, 85, 89, 90
somnolence, 85
South Africa, xii, 163, 164, 165, 167
South America, 142, 157, 159, 160
specialists, 59, 99, 106, 111, 113, 173
species, 142, 143, 158
specific phobia, 94
stability, 76, 109
stabilization, 75, 80, 82, 83, 85, 87, 90
stabilizers, 80, 82, 83
Stevens-Johnson syndrome, 24
stimulant, 6, 16, 21, 22, 24, 26, 52, 53, 46, 48, 54, 55, 68, 83, 90
stimulation, 14, 15, 62, 143
stomach, 85, 94, 112, 149, 154
street drugs, 16
stress, 19, 46, 86, 91, 102, 140
stressful events, 97
strychnine, 4
substance abuse, 11, 16, 19, 30, 53
substance use, 21, 33, 34, 63, 65, 97, 171, 181
substance use disorders(SUD), 18, 34, 63, 65, 171
substance/medication-induced anxiety disorder, 96
suicidal behavior, 77, 88
suicidal ideation, 67, 77, 87, 102, 112
suicide, 24, 62, 63, 65, 67, 76, 77, 120, 128, 180
suicide attempts, 76
supplementation, 27
suppression, 23
surgical intervention, 125, 126
Sweden, 140, 177
symbolism, 165
symmetry, 108, 109
symptomatic treatment, 36
symptomology, 26
syndrome, 17, 46, 47, 48, 50, 52, 55, 59, 64, 65, 66, 70, 107, 112
synergistic effect, 24
synthesis, 7

T

tachycardia, 70
talk therapy, 125, 137
target, 22, 48, 51, 86, 90, 112
teachers, 12, 13, 14, 19, 62, 98
techniques, 32, 86, 93, 100, 130, 140
temperament, 79, 89, 97
temporal lobe, 47, 52
tension, 96, 108, 151, 152
testing, 35, 49, 100, 108, 111, 129
textbook(s), 5, 14, 103, 156, 174, 180
therapeutic effect(s), 90, 147
therapeutic interventions, 11, 37, 41
therapist, 54, 73, 135, 138
therapy, 53, 67, 71, 80, 83, 85, 86, 87, 92, 100, 102, 103, 110, 111, 124, 135, 137, 138, 160, 180
thoughts, 42, 52, 60, 75, 77, 78, 86, 91, 98, 99, 102, 106, 109, 135, 137, 146, 153, 154, 155
threatening behavior, 63
thrombocytopenia, 81
thyroid, 71, 85, 98
thyroid stimulating hormone (TSH), 85
tic disorder, 18, 50, 54
tics, 23, 24, 54, 55, 108, 110, 113
tissue, 151
tobacco, 38, 107, 144, 147, 153
touch therapy, 124, 135, 137, 138
toxic effect, 5, 136, 137
toxic substances, 14
toxicology, 160
transformation, 142, 173
transgression, 145
traumatic brain injury (TBI), 47, 51, 55, 56
trial, 27, 52, 53, 54, 57, 71, 81, 83, 86, 87, 90, 92, 102, 112, 113, 115, 122, 130, 131, 136, 139, 140
trichotillomania, 96, 106, 108
tricyclic antidepressant(s), 21, 100, 113, 115

U

United Kingdom, 140, 177
United States, 3, 7, 11, 29, 41, 56, 59, 72, 75, 93, 105, 130, 139, 172, 174, 177

unspecified anxiety disorder, 96
unwanted thoughts, 106
upper respiratory infection, 110

V

vaccine, 5, 128, 132
variety of domains, 108
Venezuela, 160
venlafaxine, 21, 24, 68, 100, 101, 102
Venlafaxine XR, 101
victims, 33, 164
video games, 44, 56
violence, 31, 32, 33, 41, 43, 44, 56, 57, 164, 167
violent behavior, 36, 37, 57
visions, 153, 154, 155
vomiting, 82, 142, 149, 152, 153

W

Washington, 38, 57, 72, 88, 89, 93, 103, 105, 114, 130, 132, 139
weight gain, 35, 60, 81, 82, 84, 102
weight loss, 60, 84

weight management, 84
welfare, 172, 175
well-being, 48, 65, 172
willow leaf, 6
windows, 32
withdrawal, 17, 46, 48, 62, 63, 65, 66, 72, 96, 99, 102, 111
withdrawal symptoms, 102
working memory, 79
World Health Organization (WHO), xi, 119, 120, 121, 122, 123, 124, 125, 128, 129, 131, 132, 133, 166
worldview, xi, 67, 117
worldwide, 25, 125, 129

Y

young adults, 4, 13, 16, 26, 47, 63, 67, 173, 174
young people, 16, 37, 48, 49, 62, 65, 164
youth transition, 97

Z

ziprasidone, 80, 89